Sleep and its Disorders in Children and Adolescents with a Neurodevelopmental Disorder

A Review and Clinical Guide

Sleep and its Disorders in Children and Adolescents with a Neurodevelopmental Disorder

A Review and Clinical Guide

Professor Gregory Stores MD MA FRCPsych FRCP

Emeritus Professor of Developmental Neuropsychiatry, Department of Psychiatry,
University of Oxford, Oxford, UK

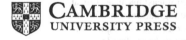
CAMBRIDGE
UNIVERSITY PRESS

CAMBRIDGE
UNIVERSITY PRESS

University Printing House, Cambridge CB2 8BS, United Kingdom

One Liberty Plaza, 20th Floor, New York, NY 10006, USA

477 Williamstown Road, Port Melbourne, VIC 3207, Australia

314-321, 3rd Floor, Plot 3, Splendor Forum, Jasola District Centre, New Delhi - 110025, India

103 Penang Road, #05-06/07, Visioncrest Commercial, Singapore 238467

Cambridge University Press is part of the University of Cambridge.

It furthers the University's mission by disseminating knowledge in the pursuit of
education, learning and research at the highest international levels of excellence.

www.cambridge.org
Information on this title: www.cambridge.org/9781107402201

First published 2014

A catalogue record for this publication is available from the British Library

Library of Congress Cataloging in Publication data
Stores, Gregory, author.
Sleep and its disorders in children and adolescents with a neurodevelopmental disorder : a review
and clinical guide / Professor Gregory Stores.
    p. ; cm.
Includes bibliographical references and index.
ISBN 978-1-107-40220-1 (paperback)
I. Title.
[DNLM: 1. Sleep Disorders – aetiology – Review.   2. Sleep Disorders – therapy –
Review.   3. Adolescent.   4. Child.   5. Mental Disorders – complications – Review.
6. Nervous System Diseases – complications – Review.   7. Sleep – physiology – Review.   WL 108]
RJ506.S55
618.92´8498–dc23

                                                                                        2014010483

ISBN 978-1-107-40220-1 Paperback

....

This book is dedicated to my wife, Christina, for her constant support and encouragement, my parents to whom I owe so much, and my children Adrian, Rebecca, Rachel and Alasdair whose characters and many accomplishments make me very proud.

Thank you to Rachel Stores and Lisa Walker who contributed to the preparation of the manuscript.

I also wish to express my gratitude to Professor Michael Gelder for the support and encouragement that he has given to me throughout my time in Oxford.

Contents

Introductory remarks

Historical perspectives

The first English textbook of paediatrics, *The Boke of Chyldren*, was published in the mid-sixteenth century. The author was Thomas Phaire, a lawyer and physician, who wished to draw attention (in fanciful terms by modern standards) to the clinical features, supposed causes, and recommended treatments of various '*infirmities of children*':

Although (as affirmeth Plinie) there are innumerable passions & diseases, where unto the bodye of man is subiecte, and as well maye chaunce in the young as in the olde: Yet for moste commonly the tender age of children is chefely vexed and greuved with these diseases folowyng (Phaire, 1545).

He then lists 40 such conditions which include neurological problems such as '*Swellyng of the head*', '*The fallying euill*' (epilepsy), '*The palsy*' and '*Gogle-eyes*' (squint). He also discussed the following sleep disturbances: '*watchyng out of measure*' (sleeplessness or insomnia), '*terryble dreames and feare in the slepe*' and '*pyssyng in bedde*'. In course of considering '*watchyng out of measure*' he stressed the importance of sleep:

Slepe is the nourishment & foode of a sucking child, and asmuch requisite as ye very teate, wherefore wha It is depruiued of the naturall rest, all the hole body falleth in distēper [ill-health or disease].

In addition to his many other high-level accomplishments, Thomas Willis, the seventeenth-century physician and anatomist (who invented the word '*neurologia*' and is credited with being the founder of clinical neuroscience), provided more extensive and detailed accounts of many childhood neurological conditions including various neurodevelopmental disorders.

However, the validity of Willis's accounts of pathophysiology and treatment is tempered by the highly speculative contemporary notions such as the humoral theory of disease which had persisted from ancient times, and 'iatrochemistry' (the theory that disease is the result of chemical reactions involving, for example, '*explosions*', '*explosive particles*' or '*spirits*', and that treatments could be chemical in type) (Williams, 2003). The curious nature of his suggested treatments rivalled Phaire's. For instance, he considered that the aims of treatment for limited intelligence were to

purifie and vollatize the Blood and nervous Liquor, together with the Animal Spirits: and also that they may clarifie the Brain and render it more Diaphanous (Willis, 1685, quoted Williams, 2003 p 358).

That said, Willis anticipated modern views about the aetiology of many disorders including intellectual disability, concerning which he distinguished between inherited, congenital and acquired causes of 'stupidity', differentiating this from 'folly' by which he seems to have meant psychiatric disorder (Williams, 2002). One of the many topics on which he lectured and wrote in his book *The London Practice of Physick* was sleep, and he is credited with making early observations of various sleep problems and disorders such as insomnia, nightmares, sleepwalking and even restless legs syndrome (Thorpy, 2000).

Needless to say, concepts, diagnostic methods and treatments have improved since the days of Phaire and Willis who, nevertheless, were well ahead of their time in some respects. Only relatively recently, paediatrics has gradually and sporadically emerged as a branch of medicine in its own right (Still, 1931). Even closer to the present day, as Millichap and Millichap (2009) have described, child neurology has developed to include the subspecialty of neurodevelopmental disability (Painter *et al.*, 2001).

The field of neurodevelopmental disorders has expanded rapidly in recent years with increasing numbers of reports from studies involving many disciplines and medical specialties. This book is concerned with a relatively neglected aspect of the predicament of very many children with a neurodevelopmental disorder, namely, sleep disturbance which can have serious harmful effects on both the child and his family.

It is inappropriate to generalize about sleep disturbance in children with neurodevelopmental disorders because of the many types of sleep disturbance now described and also the wide range of such disorders. For clinical purposes and also research, it is important to avoid reference to 'mixed groups of children with a mental handicap', which characterized many earlier sleep studies, and to consider precisely defined sleep disorders in specific subgroups of affected children.

Educational issues

Much knowledge about sleep and its disorders has accumulated in recent times but it remains under-utilized because awareness of these advances by both the general public and professionals remains inadequate. This is especially so regarding aspects of sleep and its disorders in children and adolescents.

Health education for parents and prospective parents often pays little regard to sleep. With some commendable exceptions, medical students, specialist trainees (including paediatricians and child psychiatrists, health visitors, child psychologists, and teachers) receive little relevant instruction despite the fact that all come in contact with many young people whose sleep is disturbed, sometimes with serious consequences.

Understanding of children's sleep problems has improved considerably, certainly since the time of Phaire and Willis, and clinically valuable books are now available, but the attention paid to such problems still tends to lag behind that regarding sleep disturbance in adults. However, a positive sign is that the recent revision of the *International Classification of Sleep Disorders* or ICSD-3 (American Academy of

Sleep Medicine, 2014) has improved on previous classification schemes by making paediatric aspects an integral part of its accounts of diagnostic issues.

Unfortunately, unlike nutrition and other aspects of basic health care, the topic of sleep and its disorders is neglected in both public health education and professional teaching and training (Colten & Altevogt, 2006). The extent of this neglect can be said to be striking.

Parents would benefit from knowing at least the fundamental facts about sleep, the ways in which it can be disturbed and the effects of this, as well as that, at any age, sleep problems can often be solved or, indeed, prevented (Owens et al., 2011). Rather than trying to accommodate to their children's troublesome sleep, parents would benefit from knowing that unresolved sleep issues can lead to significant learning and behavioural difficulties. Schools do not cover the subject, and teenagers rarely have advice about their sleep despite the frequency with which it is disturbed, with the potentially serious harmful effects discussed later. Consequences of this neglect include parents omitting to mention their children's sleep problems to their doctor, and failing to seek help even for extreme sleep disturbance because they think that the problem is inevitable and cannot be treated (Schreck & Richdale, 2011).

As for professional neglect, it has been found consistently that the amount of time devoted to sleep and its disorders in undergraduate medical student courses is very limited (Peile, 2010). With few exceptions, the situation seems very largely to have remained the same in more recent times and there is little reason to believe that these deficiencies have been made up significantly in higher training. As a result, sleep problems may be overlooked in primary care (Blunden et al., 2004), and relatively few paediatricians are reported to ask about sleep problems (Chervin et al., 2001), or to possess basic knowledge about children's sleep (Owens, 2001). Consequently, many opportunities to help children with sleep problems (and their families) must inevitably continue to be missed (Wiggs & Stores, 1996). The urgent need for improved training in sleep medicine at all levels has been discussed by Strohl (2011).

A similar story can be told for other clinical groups including other medical childcare specialists and nursing staff (although some health visitors have taken the initiative and set up sleep clinics for young children and their parents), and also clinical psychologists (Meltzer et al., 2009). Teachers and educational psychologists will encounter the school problems of children and adolescents whose sleep is inadequate without necessarily realising that this can be the cause (at least in part) of their learning and behaviour problems.

As Owens (2005) emphasized in her introduction to the meeting of the 2003 International Pediatric Sleep Education Task Force, healthcare staff increasingly work with patients and their families of widely different cultural origins. It is necessary, therefore, to be sensitive to the ethnic, socio-economic and cultural context of paediatric sleep disorders regarding their definition, aetiology, recognition, significance, assessment and management, as well as the need for patient and parent educational information. Gellis (2011) has reviewed the findings in studies of the effects of socio-economic status, race and ethnicity on children's sleep.

Research and clinical practice

An inevitable consequence of this widespread educational neglect is that clinical provision for children with sleep disorders (which often needs to be multidisciplinary in nature) is frequently inadequate. Not surprisingly, research in the field of children's sleep disorders has, for the most part, been limited in both quantity and also quality. The evidence base for many aspects remains limited, often consisting of collective clinical impressions which, nevertheless, can have their value. The review by Kuhn and Elliott (2003) of various treatments for children's sleep disorders in which they graded the evidence in favour of their use, indicates that, in the light of the limited and varied quality of the published research, much remains to be accomplished before many treatments used have their evidence base firmly established. However, that does not justify therapeutic inertia, merely meaning that it is appropriate to be somewhat circumspect about the likely efficacy of treatment in the individual child if only in view of individual differences in response to the treatment chosen.

Terminology

Basic terminology in the area of childhood disability can be a source of confusion. For present purposes, 'neurodevelopmental disorder' implies an impairment of the growth and development of the central nervous system. Disorders that are neurodevelopmental in origin, or that have neurodevelopmental consequences when they occur in childhood, can be the result of various pathological processes such as genetic, metabolic, toxic or traumatic.

Childhood 'neuropsychiatric disorders' can be viewed as a subset of neurodevelopmental disorders, characteristically involving prominent psychiatric disturbance arising from neurological dysfunction the precise nature of which might be ill-defined. Children with this type of disorder generally attend child psychiatric services. Autism spectrum disorder, and attention deficit hyperactivity disorder are main examples. Other forms of neurodevelopmental disorder come more readily within the terms of reference of paediatric neurology.

Many children with a neurodevelopmental disorder have an 'intellectual disability'. This (or its equivalent 'learning disability') has been defined in the UK as a significantly reduced ability to understand new or complex information, or to learn new skills (impaired intelligence), along with a reduced ability to cope independently (impaired social functioning) (Department of Health, 2001). This definition is distinct from 'learning difficulties' which is a general term referring to difficulty learning for various reasons, medical and non-medical. In North America 'learning disability' refers to specific developmental delays such as dyslexia, dyscalculia and dysgraphia. DSM-5 has substituted 'intellectual disability' (or 'intellectual disability disorder') for 'mental retardation' and ICD-11 is likely to do the same (Harris, 2013).

The term 'special educational needs' usually refers to children who have learning disabilities that make it harder for them to learn than most children of the same age. Such children require assistance that may be educational, medical, psychiatric and/or psychological. 'Children with multiple disabilities' are defined as having two or more disabling conditions that affect learning or other important life functions. To qualify for special education services each of their disabilities must be so significant that their needs could not be met by special programmes that are designed to address one of the disabilities alone.

Structure and aim of this book

The book consists of four chapters.

Chapter 1 provides an outline of sleep and its disorders in children and adolescents, more detailed accounts of which are provided in books by Mindell and Owens (2010) and Stores (2001).

Chapter 2 considers some special considerations regarding sleep disorders in children with a neurodevelopmental disorder.

Chapter 3 reviews some comorbid conditions capable of contributing to sleep disturbance in children with a neurodevelopmental disorder.

Chapter 4 is the main part of the book. Drawing on the content of previous chapters, it consists of accounts of the sleep disturbance aspects of a range of neurodevelopmental disorders, each considered individually. The accounts are subdivided into three groups:
- neurodevelopmental syndromes
- neuropsychiatric disorders
- other neurodevelopmental disorders.

It is recommended that earlier chapters should have been consulted before Chapter 4 is consulted.

Several boxes, each with a historical/clinical theme, are included in places throughout the text.

Based on a review of the literature, this structure and content of the book aim to provide a useful reference source and clinical guide for paediatricians (including paediatric neurologists and specialists in intellectual disability), child and adolescent psychiatrists, psychologists, primary care staff, nursing staff including health visitors, and others involved with child health, welfare or education, as well as parents. This intended wide appeal illustrates the fact that a multidisciplinary approach to the sleep problems of children with a neurodevelopmental disorder is ideally required. Emphasis throughout is placed on aspects of practical clinical importance. Technical accounts of limited appeal to those who are not specialists in the sleep disorders field have been avoided.

As the book is written for non-specialists in the sleep disorders field, technical abbreviations are kept to a minimum, the main exception being in Chapter 4 where the conventional abbreviation of the name of each neurodevelopmental disorder is used. A list of abbreviations, mainly for technical terms in the sleep disorders field that appear in the text, is provided at the rear of the book as this might be helpful when the bibliography is consulted.

At times, purely for convenience, the child is referred to as 'he' or 'his' rather than the female gender. In places, 'child' or 'children' can be taken to include adolescents.

Bibliography

Selected peer-reviewed articles and chapters (and some books) are cited instead of an exhaustive literature review as this would exceed the intended purpose and scope of the book. For the same reason, detailed appraisal of individual publications was not attempted. The fine details of treatment regimes (also being beyond the scope of the book) can be found in the relevant references provided.

Because research in this area is generally limited in terms of the number of studies and sometimes their scientific quality, often conclusions and recommendations can only be provisional and necessarily subject to revision in the light of further study. Frequently, reports only raise clinical possibilities rather than established facts which, nevertheless, are important to consider in assessing and treating the individual child. Ideally, in time, sufficient findings based on well-designed research will become available to allow refinement of available evidence to more adequately guide diagnosis and treatment. Also, hopefully, the literature cited will act as a stimulus to further well-designed investigations.

American Academy of Sleep Medicine. *International Classification of Sleep Disorders*, 3rd edn. Darien IL: American Academy of Sleep Medicine 2014.

Blunden S, Lushington, K, Lorenzen B *et al.* (2004). Are sleep problems under-recognised in general practice? *Arch Dis Child*, **89**, 708–12.

Chervin RD, Archbold KH, Panahi P *et al.* (2001). Sleep problems seldom addressed at two pediatric clinics. *Pediatrics*, **107**, 1375–80.

Colten HR, Altevogt BM, eds. Chapter 3: Extent and health consequences of chronic sleep loss and sleep disorders; and Chapter 4: Functional and economic impact of sleep loss and sleep-related disorders. *Sleep Disorders and Sleep Deprivation: An Unmet Public Health Problem*. Washington DC: National Academies Press 2006. 67–209.

Department of Health. *Valuing People: A New Strategy for Learning Disability for the 21st Century*. London: Department of Health 2001.

Gellis LA. Children's sleep in the context of socioeconomic status, race and ethnicity. In: El-Sheikh M. ed. *Sleep and Development: Familial and Socio-Cultural Considerations*. New York: Oxford University Press 2011. 219–44.

Harris JC. (2013). New terminology for mental retardation in DSM-5 and ICD-11. *Curr Opin Psychiatry*, **26**, 260–2.

Kuhn BR, Elliott AJ. (2003). Treatment efficacy in behavioral pediatric sleep medicine. *J Psychosom Res*, **54**, 587–97.

Meltzer LJ, Phillips C, Mindell JA. (2009). Clinical psychology training in sleep and its disorders. *J Clin Psychol*, **65**, 305–18.

Millichap JJ, Millichap JG. (2009). Child neurology: past, present, and future: part 1: history. *Neurology*, **73**, e31–3.

Mindell JA, Owens JA. *A Clinical Guide to Pediatric Sleep. Diagnosis and Management of Sleep Problems*, 2nd edn. Philadelphia: Lipincott Williams and Wilkins 2010.

Owens JA. (2001). Introduction: culture and sleep in children. *Pediatrics*, **115** Supplement 1, 201–3.

Owens JA. (2005). The practice of pediatric sleep medicine: results of a community survey. *Pediatrics*, **108**, E51.

Owens JA, Jones C, Nash R. (2011). Caregivers' knowledge, behavior, and attitudes regarding healthy sleep in young children. *J Clin Sleep Med*, **7**, 345–50.

Painter MJ, Capute A, Accardo P. (2001). Subspecialization in the care of children with neurodevelopmental disabilities. *J Child Neurol*, **16**, 131–3.

Peile E. A commentary on sleep education. In: Cappuccio FP, Miller M, Lockley SW, eds. *Sleep, Health and Society from Aetiology to Public Health*. Oxford: Oxford University Press 2010. 412–16.

Phaire T. *The Boke of Chyldren* (1545). Translated by Neale AV, Wallis HRE. Edinburgh: Livingstone 1955.

Schreck KA, Richdale AL. (2011). Knowledge of childhood sleep: a possible variable in under or misdiagnosis of childhood sleep problems. *J Sleep Res*, **20**, 589–97.

Still GF. *The History of Paediatrics*. London: *Oxford University Press* 1931.

Stores G. *A Clinical Guide to Sleep Disorders in Children and Adolescents*. Cambridge: Cambridge University Press 2001.

Strohl KP. (2011). Sleep medicine training across the spectrum. *Chest*, **139**, 1221–31.

Thorpy MJ. Historical perspective on sleep and man. In: Culebras A, ed. *Sleep Disorders and Neurological Disease*. New York: Marcel Dekker 2000. 1–36.

Wiggs L, Stores G. (1996). Sleep problems in children with severe intellectual disabilities: what help is being given? *J Appl Res Intellect Disabil*, **9**, 160–5.

Williams AN. (2002). "Of stupidity or folly": Thomas Willis's perspective on mental retardation. *Arch Dis Child*, **87**, 555–8.

Williams AN. (2003). Thomas Willis's practice of paediatric neurology and neurodisability. *J Hist Neurosci*, **12**, 350–67.

1

General outline of sleep and its disorders in children and adolescents

Basic aspects of the neurobiology of sleep

The nature of sleep

Sleep does not simply consist of the shutdown of daytime activities. The onset of sleep, waking up, and the two distinct types of sleep described shortly all involve complex brain mechanisms the modern view of which has been described by Brown *et al.* (2012). The most fundamental clinical aspect of sleep is that it is an essential part of existence in the sense that without it survival is not possible. If kept awake continuously long-term, experimental animals undergo profound deterioration in their basic bodily processes and they die.

Lesser degrees of sleep loss, and also poor quality (broken) sleep, can have serious harmful psychological and even physical effects. Without regular periods of rest, animals are unable to function properly in many ways.

In humans and related species sleep has very distinctive characteristics compared with other states of relative inactivity. Brain activity of hibernating animals is generally depressed as part of an overall slowing of bodily processes. The same is true in coma, or when unconscious. Sleep is different. For example, it is possible to be roused from sleep but, more especially, sleep shows specific patterns of brain and other physiological activity.

Interesting inter-species differences have been described. Duration of sleep within each 24 hour period varies from about 3 hours in a horse to almost 20 hours in bats. An adult human holds a mid-way position at an average of 7–8 hours. These differences are perhaps partly explained by differing vulnerability to attack by predators, although other possible explanations have been suggested.

Humans usually sleep at night in a bed; hamsters, for example, also sleep in their beds but during the day. Some animals, such as cattle and horses, can sleep standing upright; others, such as leopards, may sleep in a tree. Dolphins, and some other sea-dwelling mammals which need to be awake enough to breathe intermittently at the surface, and some other species, sleep in one half of their brain at a time, switching from one hemisphere to the other at intervals of minutes to hours ('inter-hemispheric sleep'). Roosting birds are able to sleep while maintaining their balance on a perch. Fish and reptiles also sleep or, at least, rest regularly in a way similar to sleep.

The functions of sleep

As already mentioned, sleep is necessary for survival. Sleep can also be seen as particularly important as adult human beings spend about one-third of their life asleep and children much more than that. By early school age the average child has spent more time asleep than eating, playing, exploring his environment or interacting with others.

There has been much debate about the function of sleep. Clearly, there is no single explanation. Sleep serves many different, related functions, the balance between them changing during the course of development and possibly varying from one species to another.

Different theories have emphasized mental and bodily restoration and recovery during sleep, or the laying down of memories in the brain so that learning from experience is possible. Others have speculated that dreaming is essential for the working out of possibly deep-seated emotional problems and conflicts. On the physical side, basic functions requiring adequate sleep include growth, resistance to infection and possibly the process of repair following injury or other damage to body tissues, and various other metabolic processes. Inadequate or poor quality sleep in humans can cause potentially profound psychological and physical changes which can be reversed if sleep is restored to normal.

Types of sleep

There are two very different types of sleep: non-rapid eye movement (NREM) sleep and rapid eye movement (REM) sleep. It seems that a balance between these two types is required to function well.

NREM sleep

In adults this type of sleep makes up about 75% of sleep. It is divided into four levels of increasing depth, called stages, each of which has its own characteristic brain activity as recorded by the electroencephalogram (EEG). Stages 1 and 2 are relatively light sleep; stages 3 and 4 are deep sleep from which it is especially difficult to waken. Most deep sleep (also called slow wave sleep) occurs in the first 3 hours of overnight sleep. At this depth of sleep sleepwalking and related disorders occur. Fragments of dreams can occur in NREM sleep.

REM sleep

Needless to say, the main feature of REM sleep that makes it different from NREM sleep is prominent eye movements. Because most dreaming occurs during this type of sleep, it is also called 'dreaming sleep'. Compared with the 25% by age 2 and afterwards, REM sleep takes up at least 50% of sleep in newborns (and more than this before birth) suggesting that it is particularly important for early brain development. It appears to play some part in memory although the details are unclear. In infants, 'active' sleep is the precursor of REM sleep and 'quiet' sleep is the precursor of NREM sleep. Otherwise, sleep at this age is of 'indeterminate' type.

At any age, the level of brain activity in REM sleep is high. Blood flow through the brain is increased compared with NREM sleep. EEG traces are similar to those recorded in the awake and alert state and yet skeletal musculature is effectively paralysed. This physiological contrast has led to REM sleep also being called 'paradoxical sleep' compared with 'orthodox sleep' for NREM sleep. Also, heart rate and breathing tend to be less regular in REM sleep.

Dreaming

Possibly everyone dreams, but only some can recall their dreams. Even blind people dream although without any visual imagery if they have been blind from birth or from a very early age. Often the content of dreams is a mixture of fragments of recent experiences or preoccupations but sometimes children or adults have recurrent upsetting dreams with a consistent theme based on distressing past experiences. Nightmares are particularly frightening dreams which, being related to REM sleep (which mainly occurs later in overnight sleep), also tend to occur later in the night. Dream-like experiences can occur when drifting off to sleep or in a drowsy state before waking up properly.

Pattern of overnight sleep

As illustrated in Figure 1, which shows the pattern of overnight sleep stages in a healthy child, periods of NREM and REM sleep alternate with each other several times throughout the night.

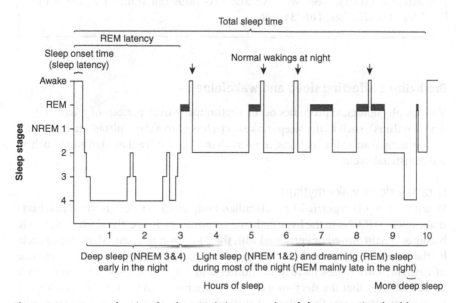

Figure 1 Hypnogram showing the characteristic progression of sleep stages in a healthy school-aged child. Reproduced from Stores (2006a).

Ideally, a short while after settling into bed, drowsiness is followed by progressively deeper levels of NREM sleep. A period of deep NREM sleep lasting 2–3 hours is then followed by a brief first period of REM sleep. The rest of the night consists of alternating periods of light NREM sleep and increasingly longer REM sleep periods, in children possibly ending with more deep sleep before they finally wake up. It is normal for anyone to wake briefly during the night, perhaps several times, although this may not be remembered. A problem only arises if it is difficult to get back to sleep at these times.

Box 1 First and second sleeps

On the basis of literary, historical and other sources, it has been claimed that, earlier in history, the norm (at least in adults) was a pattern of 'segmented', 'divided' or 'bi-modal' sleep rather than the period of uninterrupted night-time sleep which nowadays is considered to be the ideal and without which there might be concern. A 'first sleep' lasting 3–4 hours was followed spontaneously by 2–3 hours of wakefulness and then a 'second sleep' until morning. When awake, people could be active in various ways such as reading, praying, chatting or having sex. This 'natural' pattern is said to have died out, possibly from the seventeenth century, for a number of reasons such as the advent of artificial street and domestic lighting. Childhood aspects of this segmented sleep phenomenon seem to have been discussed hardly at all.

Ekirch AR. (2001). Sleep we have lost: pre-industrial slumber in the British Isles. *Am Hist Rev*, **106**, 343–86.

Biorhythms affecting sleep and wakefulness

Various physiological processes occur rhythmically over periods of a day ('circadian' rhythms), such as the sleep–wake cycle; less than a day ('ultradian' rhythms), such as temperature fluctuations; or more than a day ('infradian' rhythms), such as the menstrual cycle.

Circadian sleep–wake rhythms
When we sleep is regulated by a circadian body clock located in the suprachiasmatic nucleus (SCN) in the hypothalamus. From an early age, the sleep–wake cycle becomes synchronized or entrained with the 24 hour night–day (dark–light) cycle by the influence of external cues ('zeitgebers'), the main one being the experience of daylight. Other cues include mealtimes and social activities. The body clock usually ensures that the sleep–wake cycle is synchronized with the fluctuations in body temperature and the output of cortisol. For example, body temperature falls during overnight sleep, being lowest in deep NREM sleep.

The suprachiasmatic nucleus is acted upon by the hormone melatonin, mainly produced in the pineal gland during darkness ('the hormone of darkness') and suppressed by bright light. Therefore, melatonin promotes sleep during the night, and its suppression by daylight encourages wakefulness. It has circadian sleep–wake phase-shifting properties as well as its sleep-promoting properties. Synthetic melatonin has been used to treat some sleep disorders in adults and also children including those with neurodevelopmental disorders.

There is increasing interest in melopsin-containing 'photosensitive ganglion cells', a third type of retinal photoreceptor in addition to rods and cones. They are sensitive to environmental brightness and convey important information to the SCN. Thereby they are involved in the release of melatonin and the synchronization of circadian rhythms to the 24 hour light–dark cycle even in profoundly blind people with no rod and cone function (Foster, 2004).

Problems arise when the various circadian rhythms become uncoupled (as in jet lag, or night shift work disorder) resulting in disruption of sleep with adverse effects on daytime function and well-being. People with circadian rhythm sleep disorders are unable to sleep and wake at the times required for normal work, school and social needs. Circadian sleep–wake rhythms also vary at different ages. The body clock change that occurs at puberty is important in explaining the sleep problems that are particularly common in adolescents. At this stage of development there is a tendency for the sleep phase to shift later than at an earlier age. This causes difficulty getting to sleep and, as a result, insufficient sleep may well have been obtained by the time it is necessary to get up for school, college or work. This condition is called the 'delayed sleep–wake phase disorder' (see later). Attempts to correct the adverse effects on daytime functioning of this pubertal shift in the timing of the sleep phase (resulting in inadequate sleep) by delaying school start times are reported to improve adolescents' sleep, mood and educational attainments (Owens *et al.*, 2010). However, the feasibility of this practice is limited.

An opposite shift (i.e. to earlier onset of sleep) occurs mainly in old age when early bedtime may mean waking in the early hours because the amount of sleep required has been obtained by that time ('advanced sleep–wake phase disorder'). This 'early morning waking' in older people should not be misinterpreted as a sign of depression in which early waking is associated with impaired sleep. Something similar can happen in children who have habitually been put to bed particularly early and have soon gone to sleep. Gradually delaying the child's bedtime can help to overcome this problem.

'Irregular sleep–wake rhythm disorder', consisting of a chronic or recurrent pattern of irregular sleep and wake episodes throughout the 24 hour period, is seen in neurodegenerative disorders and some childhood neurodevelopmental disorders (see Chapter 4). 'Non-24 hour sleep–wake rhythm disorder', mainly seen in totally blind people, occurs when the intrinsic circadian pacemaker is not entrained to a 24 hour light–dark cycle (see Chapter 3).

Ultradian rhythms

Alertness and degree of sleepiness varies within each 24 hours. Generally, we are most alert in the evening before the onset of sleepiness which, therefore, might be the best time to study. Parents should avoid putting their child to bed too early i.e. during this period, because he will be unable to sleep as distinct from refusing to settle. The tendency to sleep is greatest in the early hours of the morning at the time of deep NREM sleep. Trying to work then is difficult and mistakes (including driving accidents) may well occur. To a lesser extent, sleepiness increases in the early afternoon (the 'post-lunch dip'). Use is made of this in countries where having a siesta is the rule.

The timing of the different levels of alertness and sleepiness can be different from one person to another (including children). From an early age, some individuals wake up about 2 hours earlier than most others and are very alert in the morning, but then tire early in the evening. These are so-called 'morning types' or 'larks'. Others tend to wake relatively late and have difficulty getting going in the morning but become alert and active in the evening, perhaps until quite late ('evening types' or 'owls'). Larks can have special difficulty coping with night shift work because they are required to be active when their body clock is telling them to sleep.

Changes in sleep during childhood and adolescence

Significant developmental changes in sleep occur during early life. Most obvious is the amount of sleep required for satisfactory function during the day. This is clear from Table 1 which shows the average amount of sleep that has been said to be needed for satisfactory daytime functioning at different ages, although the evidence base for such figures has been questioned (Matricciani *et al.*, 2013). Be that as it may, everyday experience indicates that children (like other age groups) vary in the amount of restorative sleep they seem to need.

- Studies of *premature babies* show that prolonged sleep (up to 20 hours a day) begins well before birth.
- *Full-term babies* sleep something like 17 hours, at least 50% taking the form of 'active' or REM-type sleep as mentioned earlier. As a result, they tend to wake more often and more readily than at an earlier age. Infants tend to pass directly into REM sleep when they fall asleep.

Table 1 Average sleep requirements at different ages in childhood and adolescence

Full-term birth	16–18 hours
1 year	15 hours
2 years	13–14 hours
4 years	12 hours
10 years	8–10 hours
Puberty	9 hours

- The circadian body clock takes time to develop but, because their body clock is not yet fully developed, *young babies'* sleep–wake pattern is so irregular that they have to be fed repeatedly during the night. However, from about 6 months, their nighttime sleep should be fairly continuous without the need for repeated feeds at night, allowing their parents to sleep.
- *By the end of the first year,* most children sleep about 15 hours a day, and daytime naps (originally taking up perhaps half of the total sleep time) should have started to reduce significantly until by about 3–4 years of age they have stopped in most children.
- Through the *toddler stage and later,* sleep requirements gradually lessen until in later childhood (before puberty) most children need about 10 hours sleep each night. Sleep tends to be particularly sound at this age.
- About the time of *puberty* the need for sleep plateaus or might actually increase compared with previously. A pubertal delay in the timing of the sleep phase also occurs at this time, making it difficult to get to sleep until later than before. This change, combined with late-night study or social activities, is likely to lead to insufficient sleep. As discussed later, most teenagers need at least 9 hours sleep (many obtain much less) without which they are at risk of various problems.

Characteristic features of sleep and its disorders in children compared with adults

The literature on sleep disturbance in adults cannot be drawn on freely when considering children and adolescents as there are many changes that take place before adulthood is reached.

- *Changes in sleep physiology* during child development have been described already.
- The *pattern of sleep disorders* is different from adults. Some sleep disorders occur much more commonly in children and adolescents, notably bedtime settling and troublesome night-waking in young children. Other examples (see later for details) include rhythmic movement disorders (such as head-banging), nocturnal enuresis, arousal disorders and delayed sleep phase syndrome especially in adolescents. Some sleep disorders previously thought to occur mainly or exclusively in adults are now recognized in children such as restless legs syndrome, periodic limb movements in sleep and REM sleep behaviour disorder.
- As discussed in Chapter 2, in the *aetiology* of children's sleep disturbance parenting practices play a major part. Parental knowledge, attitudes and emotional state often determine whether a child's sleep pattern is a problem or not. There is some evidence that mothers' attitudes and convictions (based on experience of their own early mother–child relationships) can impair their parenting competence, leading to sleep problems in their infants (Morrell, 1999). Some parents construe normal behaviour as a problem; others do not seek help when they should do so.

- *Clinical associations and manifestations.* Whereas obesity is the main cause of obstructive sleep apnoea (OSA) in adults, enlarged tonsils and adenoids are usually responsible for this sleep disorder in children, although increasingly obesity is also an important factor at this age. Periods of partial airway obstruction with hypoventilation are often seen in children with OSA rather than the discrete obstructive apnoeas which occur in adults. Also, adult OSA generally causes sleepiness and reduced activity. In contrast (as in other causes of excessive sleepiness), some children who are sleep deprived are abnormally active. This can lead to a diagnosis of attention deficit hyperactivity disorder and inappropriate treatment with stimulant drugs.
- *Significance.* Many childhood sleep disorders can be expected to resolve spontaneously in a way that is unusual in adults. That said, in the meantime (as at any age), sleep disturbance can have harmful effects (see later). However, children's sleep disorders are generally less associated with psychiatric illness than in adults. It is important for parents to know that unusual sleep-related behaviour (for example, headbanging or sleep terrors) rarely means that their child has a psychiatric or medical disorder.
- *Treatment and prognosis.* In principle, treatment of most children's sleep disorders is straightforward and likely to be effective if appropriately selected and implemented with conviction. However, parents can be unaware of simple ways in which sleep problems in children can be prevented or minimized by the way they deal with their child at bedtime or during the night. Especially in the treatment of insomnia, medication has even less a part to play in children than it has in adults. In general, behavioural methods (also often important for adults) are much more appropriate and effective. Some sleep disorders, notably arousal disorders, such as sleepwalking, usually remit spontaneously.
- The need for *multidisciplinary involvement* in assessment and management of children with disturbed sleep can be greater than in the case of adults. In addition to medical specialties, developmental psychology and child and family psychiatry often have important contributions to make.

Effects on child development of persistently disturbed sleep

There are potentially serious and widespread consequences if a child persistently fails to obtain sufficient sleep or the quality of his sleep is impaired.
- There are many ways in which *emotional state and behaviour* can be affected (Gregory & Sadeh, 2012). For example, over-tired children are often irritable, distressed and even aggressive, much to the exasperation of their parents. Sometimes such problems are frequent and seriously disrupt family life. Certain children diagnosed as having attention deficit hyperactivity disorder may well have a primary sleep disorder for which stimulant drugs are not appropriate and might make matters worse by increasing the sleeping difficulty (see Chapter 4).

Other examples include the following. Bedtime can become distressing if associated with upsetting experiences such as nighttime fears. Delayed sleep–wake phase disorder can lead to mood and other emotional changes both directly because of sleep deprivation and via the psycho-social consequences of the condition.

- *Intellectual function and education.* There is convincing evidence that inadequate and poor quality sleep can cause impaired concentration, memory, decision making and general ability to learn in children and adolescents (Dewald *et al.* 2010, Carskadon, 2011).

- *Physical effects.* Increasingly various physical disorders associated with disturbed sleep are being described (Smalldone *et al.* 2007; Spruyt *et al.* 2011; Shochat *et al.* 2014)). For example, as the production of growth hormone is closely linked to deep NREM sleep, disruption of sleep reducing the amount of this type of sleep may affect physical growth. Early onset OSA, which can impair the depth and quality of sleep, may cause some young children to fail to thrive. Persistent sleep loss in particular has been linked in adults and children with physical ill-health such as impaired immunity, obesity, hypertension and diabetes.

- *Family and other social effects* (Meltzer & Mindell, 2007, Smaldone *et al.* 2007). Parents may disagree with each other about ways of dealing with the child's refusal to go to sleep at the required time, or his insistence on joining them in their own bed after waking during the night. Because of their own loss of sleep, parents (mainly mothers) may become anxious and depressed and unable to cope (sometimes even resorting to an increased use of physical punishment) and marital relationships can become seriously strained. A child's poor sleep may affect interpersonal problems beyond his family. Irritable, difficult or otherwise disturbed behaviour is likely to affect friendships. Relationships with teachers can also suffer, especially if they are unaware that behavioural problems can be the result of inadequate or otherwise disturbed sleep.

Childhood sleep disturbance can continue into adult life

In many instances, sleep disturbance will persist beyond childhood, especially if untreated. Because of diversity of type, cause, natural history, complications and whether treated successfully or not, it is not possible to generalize across all the sleep disorders about disturbed sleep in childhood predisposing to sleep problems in adult life. Each sleep disorder has to be considered separately. The following are examples (further details of their nature are discussed later).

- *Rhythmic movement disorders* (such as headbanging) usually remit spontaneously by about 3 years of age; arousal disorders (e.g. sleepwalking) by puberty. In a minority these disorders may persist into adulthood and possibly be more difficult to treat.

- *Obstructive sleep apnoea* can begin in early childhood. Response to treatment depends on the cause. Adenotonsillar hypertrophy (the usual cause) is treatable by surgery, but anatomically more complex causes (as in some neurodevelopmental disorders, such as Down syndrome) are more difficult to correct and, therefore, the condition may persist long-term.

- *Behavioural insomnia of childhood*, largely the result of failure to learn good sleep habits (Meltzer, 2010), will persist without successful treatment and potentially set the scene for poor sleep patterns into adult life. On the other hand, treatment (usually by behavioural methods) can be successful with no recurrence of the problem.
- In contrast, *idiopathic insomnia* (seemingly constitutional in origin) typically begins in childhood, is resistant to treatment, and may well be life-long.
- Occasional *nightmares* usually cease spontaneously by adolescence or early adulthood. However, if part of post-traumatic stress disorder, they can be frequent and might persist for long periods of time.
- *Narcolepsy* often begins in childhood or adolescence and may be difficult to treat satisfactorily, in which case it can continue to be a socially disabling condition well into adult life.
- Attempted treatment of *adolescent delayed sleep–wake phase disorder* can also be less than successful if the young person is unmotivated to comply for what-ever reason. Unsuccessfully treated, the insomnia and excessive sleepiness which characterize this sleep disorder can persist long-term.

These examples are largely concerned with differences in whether or not specific childhood sleep disorders continue into adult life. However, even though the symptoms of a given sleep disorder might abate, its consequences or complications while it lasted or continues to exist can, in themselves, be a cause of disturbed sleep. Delayed sleep–wake phase disorder provides an example of this: it can lead to depression, and alcohol may be used to combat the insomnia and stimulant drugs taken to offset the daytime sleepiness. Such complications are likely, in their own right, to contribute to sleep disturbance perhaps long-term.

There are other examples of enduring sleep problems (mainly insomnia) sec-ondary to early sleep disorders which may have resolved but left a legacy of negative associations with sleeping or attempting to do so. If the original sleep disorder entailed spending long periods awake in bed, frustrated at not being able to sleep, bedtime may have become associated with being distressed rather than relaxed and ready to sleep (so-called *conditioned insomnia*). Long-lasting negative associations may develop in other ways such as having been sent to bed as punishment or experiencing night-time fears.

Prevalence of disturbed sleep in children and adolescents

Overall, from early years to adolescence, 25% or more of children in general have a significant sleep disturbance (Owens, 2008). However, as discussed in Chapters 2 and 3, prevalence rates well in excess of this are reported in certain high risk groups, namely, children with an intellectual disability, other neurodevelopmental disorder, psychiatric condition or chronic physical illness.

Aetiological factors

In explaining the cause of sleep problems at any age, both physical and psychological possibilities (perhaps in combination) have to be considered. In both children and adults, psychological, psychiatric, neurological, respiratory, metabolic, endocrine, genetic, pharmacological or other physical factors may have an influence. The following factors may play a part in the development and course of various forms of disturbed sleep. They illustrate the need for a wide-ranging assessment of the individual child.

● *Constitutional including genetic factors* can be important. For example, there is often a strong family history in children with arousal disorders (sleepwalking, sleep terrors, confusional arousals; see later).

● *Maturational factors.* In very young children a degree of early brain maturation is required for the biological clock controlling sleep–wake rhythms to develop (Mirmiran *et al.*, 2003).

● *Developmental changes in brain systems controlling sleep.* Adolescent insomnia and excessive daytime sleepiness can be the result of pubertal changes in sleep physiology combined with altered lifestyle including late-night social activities (Wolfson & Carskadon, 2003).

● *Parenting: practices* can profoundly influence any young children's sleep patterns. Lack of consistent routine, poor limit-setting and reinforcement by paying too much attention to a child's reluctance to settle to sleep can cause or maintain sleep problems. This is called *behavioural insomnia of childhood* (Meltzer, 2010) as distinct from insomnia due to other causes. The provision by parents of a physical and emotional environment conducive to their child's learning good sleep habits and maintaining satisfactory sleep comes within this same category of important factors.

● *Psychological factors.* As described in Chapter 3, a child's mental state (including psychiatric conditions) can seriously affect sleep.

● *Medical factors.* This is illustrated in the neurodevelopmental disorders that are the subject of Chapter 4. In addition, as discussed in Chapter 3, sleep can be disturbed in a variety of other medical conditions which may be comorbid with the neurodevelopmental disorder.

● Some *medications* which may be taken by children as part of their paediatric or psychiatric care can disturb sleep (Herman & Sheldon, 2005). Potential causes of insomnia include stimulant drugs for attention deficit hyperactivity disorder, pseudoephedrine, theophylline and some antidepressants. Excessive sleepiness may be caused by sedative-hypnotic drugs including benzodiazepines and some antihistamines, major tranquillizers, opioids and some anti-epileptic drugs such as barbiturates, valproate and carbamazepine. Zolpidem and some antidepressants have been linked with the occurrence of parasomnias, especially sleepwalking, although some doubt has been expressed about the strength of this association (Pressman, 2007).

- *Other substance effects.* Alcohol initially causes sleepiness but, later in the night, increased rapid eye movement sleep ('REM rebound') can cause nightmares. Features of alcohol withdrawal include insomnia which can also be the result of excessive caffeine intake and nicotine use.

Classification of sleep disorders

The general term *sleep disturbance* covers both *sleep problems* and *sleep disorders*, the difference between which must be kept clear for clinical purposes. Unfortunately, often this basic distinction is not made. *Sleep behaviour* simply means behaviour associated with sleep. It does not necessarily denote that the behaviour is problematic and, indeed, some sleep behaviours may be conducive to satisfactory sleep.

At any age, there are just three basic *sleep problems* (or complaints):

- *Insomnia* (otherwise referred to as *sleeplessness*) taking the form of not readily getting to sleep, difficulty staying asleep, and/or waking early and not returning to sleep. Sometimes unrefreshing sleep is included.
- *Excessive daytime sleepiness (hypersomnia).*
- *Parasomnias and abnormal sleep related movements.* Put simply this refers to behaving in unusual ways, having strange experiences or exhibiting unusual movements in relation to sleep.

These sleep problems are not diagnoses or conditions in their own right, no more than is 'breathlessness' or 'pain'. For the correct advice or treatment to be chosen, it is necessary to identify the underlying cause of a sleep problem, i.e. the *sleep disorder*. Attempts to treat the sleep problem without accurate diagnosis of the underlying cause are likely to be unsuccessful. Main sleep disorders underlying each of the above sleep problems are discussed in the Subsection towards the end of this chapter.

The third edition of the *International Classification of Sleep Disorders* (ICSD-3) (American Academy of Sleep Medicine, 2014) is the foremost source of information about sleep disorders. The comprehensive nature of ICSD-3 is illustrated by its various sections of sleep disorders as follows:

- Insomnia
- Sleep related breathing disorders
- Central disorders of hypersomnolence
- Circadian rhythm sleep–wake disorders
- Parasomnias
- Sleep related movement disorders
- Other sleep disorder

Appendix A: Sleep related medical and neurological disorders

Appendix B discusses the forthcoming ICD-10-CM coding for substance-induced sleep disorders.

Clinically valuable and up-to-date details concerning each diagnosis are arranged under the following headings:

- Alternate names
- Diagnostic criteria
- Essential features
- Associated features
- Clinical and pathophysiological subtypes
- Demographics
- Predisposing and precipitating factors
- Familial pattern
- Onset, course and complications
- Developmental issues
- Pathology and pathophysiology
- Polysomnographic and other objective findings
- Differential diagnosis
- Unresolved issues and further directions
- Bibliography

Specific ICD codes are listed at the beginning of each diagnosis.

There is merit in using this system of classification as it is considered to be more diagnostically specific and up-to-date than the DSM and ICD classifications of sleep disturbance. The relationship of ICSD-3 to these other classification systems is explained in its Introduction which also draws attention to differences between ICSD-3 and its 2005 precursor ICSD-2.

Box 2 Dickensian diagnoses

Charles Dickens (1812–1870) was highly accomplished in many ways, including as a clinical observer of illness and disease in which he took a special interest. He seems to have incorporated his detailed descriptions of real sufferers into many of his fictional characters both adults and children. So accurate were his descriptions (well ahead of his time) that it has been possible to discuss the possible diagnoses (in modern terms) depicted in this way. Examples of these putative diagnoses include such developmental and sleep disorders as intellectual impairment, epilepsy, autism, Tourette syndrome, OSA, sleep terrors, nightmares and restless legs syndrome.

When medicine was only just beginning to recognise the importance of physical signs, the characters in the world of Dickens's imagination are so real that they have recognisable disorders of body and mind, described with the accuracy and insight of a great clinical observer.

Sir Russell Brain (1995). Dickensian diagnoses. *BMJ*, **ii**, 1553–6.

General principles of assessment

Screening

It cannot be assumed that a child's sleep problem has already come to professional attention (Chervin *et al.*, 2001; Blunden *et al.*, 2004). Parents may not seek help for even grossly disturbed sleep patterns in the mistaken belief that it is an inevitable and untreatable problem, especially in the case of developmentally delayed children (Robinson & Richdale, 2004). For that reason, as part of developmental assessments as well as clinical history-taking in general, it is appropriate to screen all children for a sleep disturbance. Such screening should be repeated periodically as sleep disorders might arise in the course of development.

Routinely, history-taking should at least include the following basic queries:
- Bedtime difficulties or settling to sleep?
- Waking during the night?
- Breathing problems while asleep?
- Unusual behaviours, experiences or movements at night?
- Difficulty waking up in the morning?
- Being unusually sleepy or 'over-tired' during the day?

Alternatively, screening can be achieved by means of the five-item instrument called BEARS (B=bedtime issues, E=excessive daytime sleepiness, A=awakenings at night, R=regularity and duration of sleep, S=snoring) (Owens & Dalzell, 2005).

Otherwise, a somewhat fuller but still brief standardized screening questionnaire can be used. Tietze *et al.* (2012) analysed sleep questionnaires that have been used to assess children's sleep. Their use can have both strengths (especially general practicality for usual clinical purposes) but also weaknesses in that many have not been adequately evaluated psychometrically and/or they are clinically limited in scope or predictive value (Lewandowski *et al.*, 2011). There is a need for more satisfactory instruments to be developed.

The same point has been made by Spruyt and Gozal (2011) in their own comprehensive review of currently available paediatric sleep questionnaires in the light of their mainly psychometric criteria for the satisfactory design of such assessments. Although not meeting as many of these criteria as some other questionnaires, the Children's Sleep Habits Questionnaire is worth considering as a brief screening questionnaire because of the range of sleep problems that it briefly covers, and its versions for both toddlers/preschool children (Goodlin-Jones *et al.*, 2008) and school-age children (Owens *et al.*, 2000). Alternatives include the Sleep Disturbance Scale for Children (Bruni *et al.*, 1996) and the Simonds and Parraga Sleep Questionnaire (Simonds & Parraga, 1982).

Other questionnaires focus on particular aspects of sleep such as sleep disordered breathing, e.g. the Pediatric Sleep Questionnaire (Chervin *et al.* 2000), or excessive sleepiness, such as the self-report Daytime Sleepiness Scale (Drake *et al.*, 2003). Instruments for assessing sleep phase preference (chronotype) in children include the Children's Chronotype Questionnaire for use by parents (Werner *et al.*, 2009). A recently developed self-report measure of sleep patterns, sleep hygiene and sleep disturbance in school-age children (The Children's Report of Sleep Patterns) offers the prospect of providing valuable information that would not otherwise be obtained from parents' accounts alone (Meltzer *et al.*, 2013).

Although parents are necessarily the main informants about children's sleep, certain caveats are appropriate regarding the accuracy of the information obtained in this way. Parents' attitudes to their child's sleep vary. They can have different ideas of what is normal, they may be unable to cope with normal behaviour because of their emotional state, or they might misconstrue sleep disturbance as awkward behaviour e.g. by viewing pathological sleepiness as laziness or boredom. For these and other reasons, subjective and objectively derived information may not correspond with each other.

In addition to screening and assessing a child's sleep, his overall physical and psychiatric condition may merit comprehensive screening and regular review, partly to identify factors that might be contributing to his sleep disturbance. Similarly, the possibility of medication effects should be monitored.

Diagnosis of the sleep disorder

Screening for sleep symptoms simply highlights the possibility of a sleep disorder and, as already emphasized, does not constitute a diagnosis. As mentioned earlier, many sleep disorders are now officially recognized, many affecting children and adolescents.

Identification of a sleep disorder requires comprehensive clinical enquiry consisting of the following.

- *Detailed clinical history*, especially about the sleep disturbance. Naturally, parents are the main source of information but the child or siblings may be able to make useful additions. Enquiries may also be extended to teachers if appropriate. This collective information, ideally incorporating fine detail of the nature of the sleep disturbance (i.e. its start, development and current pattern), should include factors which predispose, precipitate and maintain the problem.
- *Review of the child's 24 hour sleep–wake pattern and parenting practices* including those related to sleep hygiene (see later). Table 2 suggests a scheme for achieving this, bearing in mind the possibility of day-to-day variations and differences between weekdays and weekends.

Table 2 Review of child's 24 hour sleep–wake pattern (modified according to child's age)

Evening
What time is the child's last meal?
What activities typically take place between then and getting ready for bed?
Does the child take any sleep medicine?

Going to bed
Who gets the child ready for bed and how? Is it always the same person and done in the same way?

Table 2 (cont.)

Is there a bedtime routine? If so, what is the sequence of events? Does it include a wind-down period?

What time does he go to bed?

Is he put to bed awake or asleep?

Does he fall asleep in the same environment as he will experience when he wakes in the night?

Where and how does he fall asleep (own bed, parent's bed, downstairs, being rocked, nursed or fed, with or without a parent present)?

Does he need a bottle, dummy or special object to fall asleep or want someone else to sleep with?

Does he express fears about going to bed?

Does he have his own room?

Is the bedroom conducive to sleep or is it a place for entertainment or other arousing experiences?

Does he have any unusual experiences when going off to sleep?

Exactly what happens if the child will not go to bed or does not go to sleep readily? Who deals with the problem and how consistently?

Night-time

Does the child wake during the night? If so when, and how often? Does he get up in the night to go to the toilet or to have a drink? Is he able to return to sleep easily or does he need his parents or join them in their bed? If so, what precisely happens, who is involved and what is the result?

Is the child's sleep disturbed in other ways, e.g. restlessness, sleeptalking, sleepwalking, headbanging or rocking, teeth grinding, nightmares or terrified episodes, jerking or convulsive movements or other episodes of disturbed behaviour? How often do these things occur, what time of night, how long do they last and does he seem awake at the time? What do the parents do?

Does the child snore or have any difficulty breathing when asleep?

Does he wet the bed?

Waking

What time does the child wake up? For how long has he slept?

Does he wake up spontaneously or have to be woken? Is it very difficult to wake him up?

Does he look tired? Is he irritable and in a bad mood?

Does he have any unusual experiences and how does he feel between waking up and getting out of bed?

Daytime

Is the child drowsy or does he sleep during the day? If he sleeps, can he resist doing so and does he fall asleep when engaged in activities?

What is the number, duration and timing of naps?

What is the total time asleep each 24 hours?

Do his muscles become weak when he laughs, is upset or surprised?

Does he find it difficult to concentrate?

Has his performance at school deteriorated?

Is he overactive, irritable or depressed?

Are there any other unusual episodes during the day?

From Stores, 2001

- The child's *developmental history*;
- *Family history and family circumstances*;
- Both *physical and behavioural examination* may well be appropriate;
- Possibly *further assessments*:
  - A *sleep diary*, kept for at least 2 weeks, can provide information about the pattern of sleep related events and parental activities.
  - By means of a wristwatch-type device, *actigraphy* (Meltzer & Westin, 2011) records movements which indicate overall sleep–wake patterns, without details of sleep physiology, over long periods if required. Uses include the investigation of circadian sleep–wake cycle disorders and periodic limb movements in sleep.
  - *Polysomnography* (PSG), in a sleep laboratory or by means of home recordings, provides detailed physiological information about sleep if required. Main examples include evaluation of excessive daytime sleepiness such as the diagnosis of sleep apnoea or narcolepsy, and for the diagnosis of parasomnias where their nature is unclear from the clinical details, the episodes are unusual or there may be more than one type of parasomnia or another form of sleep disorder.
  - The Multiple Sleep Latency Test, involving daytime PSG, is an objective measure of sleepiness. Basic PSG may be extended to include respiratory recording (including oximetry) for the investigation of sleep disordered breathing, or additional electroencephalography channels if epilepsy is being considered.
  - *Audiovisual recordings*, used at home (by means of parents' own equipment) or in hospital, can provide more accurate information than descriptions of nighttime occurrences provided in clinic.
  - *Other laboratory tests*, as indicated, such as levels of hypocretin if narcolepsy is suspected.

Referral for assessment at a specialist paediatric service (such as ENT in the case of OSA) or a sleep disorders clinic might be required for accurate diagnosis in difficult or complicated cases.

Basic treatment principles

Just as there are many sleep disorders, a wide range of treatment options is available from which a choice can be made depending on the child's type of sleep disorder. It is worth re-emphasizing that treatment of a sleep disturbance must be preceded by diagnosis of the underlying cause, with an attempt to identify factors which predispose to, precipitate and maintain the sleep disturbance.

The evidence base for the treatments currently recommended needs to be improved by more high-quality research (Kuhn & Elliott, 2003; Brown *et al.*, 2013). In the meantime, however, in addition to the findings of the methodologically sound studies that are available, opinions of respected authorities based on clinical experience can also provide important guidance concerning the management of individual children.

General aspects

- *Education of parents* (and children themselves if appropriate) is important concerning the developmental importance of sleep, how to promote good sleep habits from an early age, and also an understanding of realistic expectations at different ages. An optimistic view of treatment possibilities should be encouraged and the chosen treatment should be acceptable to the parents and within their capabilities. Help and support may be required to ensure persistence in implementing the treatment, especially as the sleep problem (e.g. bedtime resistance or night-time crying) may worsen before it improves.

  In addition to the accurate identification of sleep disorders and the correct choice of treatment, success (hopefully shown to be long-lasting) will depend on parents' preference, capabilities and commitment, the child's willingness and ability to comply, and an adequate trial of treatment which sometimes enquiry reveals to be lacking.

- Basic principles of *sleep hygiene* help to promote good sleep habits (Jan *et al.*, 2008). These can be sufficient in themselves in preventing or treating disturbed sleep (especially insomnia) but are also useful as an accompaniment of more specific treatment for a given sleep disorder. Aspects of good sleep hygiene (the details of which vary with the child's age) are shown in Table 3.

Table 3 Basic principles of sleep hygiene (varying with age)

Sleeping environment should be conducive to sleep
Familiar setting
Comfortable bed
Correct temperature
Darkened, quiet room
Non-stimulating
No negative associations (e.g. punishment)
Encourage
Bedtime routines
Consistent bedtime and waking up times (weekdays, weekends, holidays within reason)
Going to bed only when tired
Thinking about problems and plans before going to bed
Falling asleep without parents (young children)
Regular daily exercise, exposure to sunlight, and general fitness
Avoid
Overexcitement near bedtime
Late evening exercise
Caffeine-containing drinks late in the day
Smoking and excessive alcohol (teenagers)
Large meals late at night
Excessive or late napping during the day
Too much time awake in bed (especially if distressed)
Excessive weight gain

From Stores, 2001

Behavioural treatments

Behavioural methods (Wiggs, 2009) are often considered appropriate especially (although not only) for insomnia which is the main sleep complaint at any age. Behavioural treatments are intended to help the child to learn good sleep habits and/or unlearn inappropriate sleep behaviours. They are recommended as first-line treatment for behavioural insomnia of childhood (Meltzer, 2010). The various behavioural treatments that have been used include the following.

- *Standard extinction* (or letting the child 'cry it out') in which reinforcement of unwanted behaviour at bedtime or during the night is avoided by removal of the parents' presence and ignoring the child's demands for attention, including wanting to join his parents in their bed. This is usually an effective treatment but one which most parents cannot tolerate because they find it too distressing or they feel too guilty to persist with it.
- In *graduated extinction methods* (which most parents find more acceptable) over subsequent nights or longer they gradually reduce their physical proximity to their child or the time spent with him when he cries. In both methods, interaction with the child must be avoided.
- In the *checking method*, when the child cries the parent checks him about every 10 minutes (or less depending on the parent's preference) to briefly reassure him without doing anything else. The time period is then gradually increased.
- *Faded bedtime with response cost* involves systematically delaying bedtime to associate with falling asleep before bringing it forward gradually once the association has become established. The response cost aspect refers to being removed from bed if not asleep after a specified time.
- *Stimulus control* means reducing cues associated with being awake when in bed and increasing associations with getting to sleep including positive pre-bedtime routines.
- *Scheduled waking* treatment for night waking (assuming its timing is consistent) involves very briefly waking the child 15 minutes before the spontaneous awakening is due. The scheduled wakes are gradually phased out once the spontaneous awakenings subside.
- *General reinforcement measures* (such as star charts) can be helpful with pre-school and older children.

In the light of the limited and varied quality of the published research, according to Kuhn and Elliott (2003) extinction and graduated extinction including the checking procedure, together with parental education, can be classed as 'well-established' treatments; scheduled awakenings are 'probably efficacious'; and extinction with parental presence and faded bedtime/positive routines are 'promising'. Sleep hygiene in general has yet to be evaluated systematically.

The same authors also evaluated the use of behavioural treatments for sleep disturbances other than insomnia. They considered that, overall, although occasional attempts have been made to treat such circadian rhythm disorders as delayed sleep–wake phase disorder and irregular sleep–wake patterns, convincing empirical evidence of efficacy was limited. They classified scheduled awakenings for sleep terrors and sleepwalking as 'promising' but the evidence in favour of behavioural treatment for nightmares was felt to be more limited. The review by Brown *et al.* (2013) of sleep treatments for children with chronic health conditions (such as intellectual disability, visual impairment and some neuro-developmental disorders) suggested that research on non-pharmacological treatments was methodologically weak but that some interventions including those of a behavioural nature were promising and appropriate to use on a trial basis.

All things considered, it seems reasonable to conclude that, although formal evidence of the use of behavioural treatments for children's sleep disorders needs to be improved, it is appropriate to employ them with discretion and discernment. Various guides for parents are available such as Ferber (2013) and Quine (1997).

Pharmacological treatments

Because medication is a popular and tempting form of treatment, relatively detailed consideration here seems appropriate.

At the start of their detailed review of medication for children's sleep disorders, Pelayo and Dubik (2008) make the point that this type of treatment is widespread despite the serious lack of reliable evidence to justify its use. Medications are typically not FDA approved for specific childhood sleep disorders, and their use is generally based on extrapolation from findings in adult studies. Ideal properties of hypnotics for use with children are considered to be high oral bioavailability; short elimination half-life; rapid onset of action; once-nightly dosing; low risk for dependence, abuse, tolerance, withdrawal and rebound effects, no daytime residual effects or other side-effects; and no significant reductions in REM and NREM sleep stages. Medications currently used for children fall short of these requirements, and authors invariably emphasize the need for methodologically sophisticated research in this area. In the meantime, opinions have been offered with a note of caution.

Most discussions focus on *insomnia* as the main complaint made by parents about their child's sleep. On the basis that this problem is usually associated with behavioural factors, it is generally agreed that the evidence for efficacy is in favour of behavioural treatment in the first instance with medication having a limited part to play if necessary, possibly combined with behavioural measures.

Owens and Moturi (2009) comprehensively reviewed the pharmacological treatment of paediatric insomnia. They emphasize the potentially serious developmental effects of insomnia and the need for screening and accurate diagnosis of any sleep disorder that screening suggests. In the light of recent USA consensus group discussions (Owens *et al.*, 2005; Mindell *et al.*, 2006), indications for pharmacotherapy are considered to be

- failure of a child to respond sufficiently to behavioural treatment
- parental inability to implement behavioural methods
- possibly if the child is physically ill or in acutely stressful situations.

Contraindications include
- potential harmful interactions between the insomnia medication and other concurrent medication such as opiates, or other central nervous system depressant substances including alcohol or illicit substances
- where opportunities for follow-up or checking for side-effects are limited
- where insomnia is part of a primary sleep disorder e.g. OSA
- when inappropriate parenting practices are primarily at fault.

Other considerations emphasized by Owens and Moturi (2009) include:
- behavioural treatment being preferable to medication in the first instance, although a combination of the two might be appropriate
- choice of medication including its duration of action and timing in relation to the type of insomnia, e.g. whether it needs to be short-acting or longer
- the need to balance the likely advantage of medication against possible adverse effects
- clarifying treatment goals and expectations in consultation with parents, and ensuring adequate follow-up
- the special considerations in children with neurodevelopmental disorders including their common comorbidities (see Chapters 2 and 4).

The rest of their review covers the following groupings of pharmacological agents:
- alpha agonists including clonidine, a much-used drug for childhood insomnia despite little support for its use
- melatonin
- prescribed and over-the-counter antihistamines, the most commonly used sedative for children (Schnoes *et al.*, 2006), again despite a shortage of empirical support
- chloral hydrate and barbiturates
- benzodiazepines (with their various drawbacks including their tendency to respiratory depression worsening OSA) and benzodiazepine receptor agonists such as zolpidem
- antidepressants with sedating properties which are rarely an appropriate choice
- antipsychotics (also considered to be rarely appropriate)
- anti-epileptic drugs, some of which can improve sleep through better seizure control although others have been implicated with the development of insomnia
- various herbal supplements, the use of which in children generally lacks empirical support.

Melatonin deserves special mention because of its popularity, mainly as a treatment for childhood insomnia and perhaps especially in children with a neurodevelopmental disorder. How far it deserves this popularity is yet to be adequately clarified. As mentioned earlier, melatonin is part of the biological clock system which controls circadian sleep–wake and associated rhythms. Its secretion is regulated by the suprachiasmatic nucleus. It has both circadian sleep phase-shifting and sleep-promoting (hypnotic) properties. It has tended to be promoted for use with children despite relatively few methodologically sound studies and inconsistent findings (London New Drugs Group, 2008).

However, a number of more recent reports (to which reference is made by Owens and Moturi (2009) and Hollway and Aman (2011), with the addition of the study, for example, by Appleton *et al.* (2012)), provide more convincing evidence that melatonin can be effective, although inconsistency of response from one child to another has yet to be explained. Other important issues concern dosage, short- and long-acting forms of the drug, side-effects, other possible adverse effects and long-term efficacy. Ramelteon, a MT-1 and MT-2 melatonin receptor agonist, is currently being evaluated in childhood insomnia. It is generally considered appropriate to assess the usefulness of melatonin if behavioural treatments have been adequately tried without success.

In addition to discussing medications for insomnia, Pelayo and Dubic (2008) also considers medication for narcolepsy, OSA, restless legs syndrome and periodic limb movements in sleep. Medications can have some part to play in the primary parasomnias (see shortly), for example arousal disorders such as sleepwalking, nightmares, and rhythmic movement disorders e.g. headbanging (Kuhn & Elliott, 2003) although, again, behavioural methods may be thought appropriate in the first instance. Successful pharmacological treatment of the medical and psychiatric conditions which can give rise to secondary parasomnias can be expected to lessen this category of sleep disorder.

Other forms of treatment

- *Chronotherapy* for circadian sleep–wake cycle disorders (Raffray *et al.*, 2011) involves resetting the biological clock by progressively altering sleep–wake times to synchronize with normal daily activities and events. Alternatively, exposure to bright light (which controls melatonin output) or administration of exogenous melatonin can be helpful (Bjorvatn & Pallesen, 2009).
- *Physical methods* include adenotonsillectomy, continuous positive airway pressure and weight reduction for OSA.
- Where emotional disturbance is marked in either the child or other family members, *psychological or psychiatric help* will need to be arranged.

Subsection: Childhood sleep problems and the recognition and management of their main underlying sleep disorders

This subsection is organized in terms of the sleep disorders that might underlie the three basic sleep problems of insomnia, excessive daytime sleepiness and parasomnias/sleep related movement disorders for each of which a clinical scheme is suggested as an aid to diagnosis.

For treatment approaches, reference should be made to the general principles described earlier in this chapter. In addition, Kotagal (2012) provides further details of diagnosis and management of a range of specific sleep disorders with information about the level of evidence about the treatments mentioned.

Insomnia

Paediatric insomnia (otherwise referred to as *sleeplessness*) has been officially defined as "repeated difficulty with sleep initiation, duration, consolidation, or quality that occurs despite age-appropriate time and opportunity for sleep and results in daytime functional impairment for the child and/or family" (Owens & Moturi, 2009). In basic clinical terms, insomnia covers difficulty falling asleep, troublesome waking during the night, and waking early in the morning unable to return to sleep. The many possible causes (Lipton *et al.*, 2008) vary with the age of the child, although the following breakdown according to age should not be interpreted too strictly as there can be overlap between the different age groups. A child's developmental age can be more important than chronological age in determining his type of sleep disturbance. At any age, childhood insomnia is associated with parenting stress.

Infants
Despite the close associations between parenting practices and infant sleep (Sadeh *et al.*, 2010), ways of preventing or dealing with babies' sleep problems are rarely taught to parents (or prospective parents) many of whom, therefore, suffer needless loss of sleep and distress because their child does not sleep well. The following general guidelines for parents have been suggested to avoid bad sleep habits later on by encouraging good sleep habits from the start, although babies vary in their response to the recommendations and parents differ in their ability to adhere to them. Such advice and related issues have been discussed by St James-Roberts (2008).

- *Establish a clear difference in your baby's experience between day and night* to help to develop his body clock which controls sleep and wakefulness.
- *Do not prolong night-time feeding* beyond the age (about 6 months) when the baby's body clock has developed enough to confine feeding to daytime.
- *Teach your baby to fall asleep alone* so that when he wakes in the night (a natural occurrence at all ages) he will be able to fall asleep again without requiring your attention (*self-soothing*).
- Related to the last point, *have your baby fall asleep in the same environment as he will experience when he wakes in the night.*
- *Establish a consistent 24 hour routine*, including a bedtime routine that provides cues that it is time to go to sleep.
- *Ensure the sleeping environment is conducive to sleep.*

Risk factors for *sudden infant death syndrome (SIDS)* and their avoidance have been discussed by Fleming *et al.* (2006).

Toddlers and pre-school children
Many children of this age present a problem of recurrently not going to bed at the required time, and/or waking repeatedly at night demanding their parents' attention, including coming into their bed. Medical factors must be excluded but the usual explanation is that the child has not been taught good sleep habits (so-called

behavioural insomnia of childhood). In her account of the treatment of this problem, Meltzer (2010) emphasizes (for prevention as well as treatment) the importance of establishing from an early age a consistent bedtime and naptime appropriate for the child's age, having an enjoyable but relaxing bedtime routine which prepares him for sleep, and teaching him to fall asleep independently.

- *Bedtime problems* usually mean that the child refuses to get ready for bed, to go to bed or stay in bed. Otherwise he adopts delaying tactics about going to bed. These difficulties are best dealt with by a combination of consistent routine and equally consistently setting limits to the child's behaviour, preferably during the day as well as at bedtime. Meltzer's suggestions for limit-setting include rewarding good behaviour and ignoring bad behaviour.
- *Night waking problems* can be helped by ensuring that the child falls asleep independently in the same setting as he will experience when he wakes during the night and by having acquired from an early age the ability to fall asleep alone. Standard or graduated extinction and fading methods (see earlier) are means of treating troublesome night waking.
- *Early morning waking* can be very distressing to parents, and disruptive to the whole family if a child habitually wakes very early, does not go back to sleep and is noisy or demands attention. In preschool children, early waking can be the natural end of overnight sleep as in morning larks (described previously) or the final episode of the night waking, in which case the child may well return to sleep if his parents attend to him. Ways must be found of teaching him the difference between night and day to signal when it is appropriate to get up or not, as well as reward for not getting up too early and disturbing the family.

At this age and later, with persistence and, if necessary, support and encouragement, parents can achieve improvements in their child's sleep in a relatively short time, but they should be made aware that initially the problems may worsen before they improve.

School-age children

Some of the causes of insomnia in preschool children still apply in older children but other factors become more relevant with increasing age.

- *Night-time fears* are common from early childhood onwards (Kushnir & Sadeh, 2011). The content of the fears tends to change from aspects of the immediate environment (e.g. shadows or noises) through imaginary objects (ghosts, monsters) or the dark, to more realistic and specific fears concerning the child's own health, for example. Such fears are usually transient and require only reassurance and comfort until they cease. In some children the fears are so intense and persistent that they reach phobic proportions and need special attention.

The cause of the fear should be investigated. The night-time fear might be one aspect of an anxiety state, including post-traumatic stress disorder, in which case the child might also suffer from nightmares. The content of the fear or nightmare might be revealing, suggesting abuse, for example. Other sleep disturbances (e.g. alarming hypnagogic hallucinations) may be the cause of the night-time fears. The child's reluctance to go to bed because he or she is genuinely afraid must be distinguished from pretending to be afraid as a delaying tactic.

Behavioural treatment is said to be effective in cases of severe night-time fears. The child should be helped by learning positive associations with bedtime and by not going to bed so early that he or she lies awake in a fearful state.

- *Other worries and anxiety* about daytime matters such as school progress may cause difficulty in getting to sleep or staying asleep. Sympathetic discussion of the child's worries, attention to the source of concern if possible, and ways of helping the child to relax at night, are generally thought to help. More specific psychiatric measures will be needed if the child has an anxiety or depressive disorder, or if there is evidence of serious problems within the family.
- A child will be unable to settle to sleep if *bedtime is too early*. Like some adults and even other species, children often have an evening period of intense wakefulness and activity before they begin to relax in preparation for sleep. A child is physiologically unable to sleep if put to bed in this 'forbidden zone'. Instead the sequence of events leading up to bedtime should be arranged so that the child goes to bed when 'sleepy tired'.
- *Restless legs syndrome* (Simakajornboon *et al.*, 2009), or *Willis–Ekbom disease*, is now more described in children than formerly. The condition is highly familial. Presenting symptoms in children can be somewhat different than in adults (de Weerd *et al.*, 2013). These include a variety of disagreeable feelings ('weird', 'funny', 'wiggly' etc.) in the legs (or arms) occurring mainly when at rest and with an urge to move them in order to gain some relief. This results in difficulty getting to sleep or getting back to sleep during the night, and tiredness and sleepiness during the day. *Periodic limb movements in sleep* (see later) are a common accompaniment. When they occur around bedtime, restless legs syndrome symptoms may be diagnosed as 'growing pains'. If associated with systemic iron deficiency, treatment of restless legs syndrome with iron supplements is appropriate. Otherwise (as also in periodic limb movements in sleep), if necessary, gabapentin or, in older children, dopamine receptor antagonists might be effective.
- The original source of concern may no longer exist but the difficulty falling asleep may persist because the child has developed the habit of lying awake in bed in an agitated state *(conditioned insomnia)*.
- *Childhood onset insomnia* or *idiopathic insomnia* refers to a lifelong difficulty sleeping not attributable to environmental, emotional, or medical factors and therefore of constitutional origin. The condition is usually diagnosed retrospectively in adult life.
- *Early morning waking* (see above) may persist from an earlier age in which case the explanations include the problem being part of *advanced sleep–wake phase disorder* in which the child's bedtime and sleep onset is so early that his sleep requirements have been met well before other members of the family wake in the morning. Gradual resetting of the time the child goes to sleep is required. In older children and adolescents, early morning wakening may be part of an anxiety or depressive disorder. Otherwise, the child may have been woken too early by noise or other environmental factors which intrude into his sleep.

Adolescents

High rates of sleep problems including insomnia have been consistently (and internationally) reported in adolescents (Gradisar *et al.*, 2011). At puberty a change from the highly efficient sleep of prepubertal children to less satisfactory sleep can occur. Physiological changes at puberty together with psychosocial demands of adolescence can further conspire to disrupt sleep patterns (Crowley *et al.*, 2007) with potentially serious psychological, educational, social, and physical consequences including accidental injury (Shochat *et al.*, 2014).

- *Worries, anxiety and depression* are commonly quoted reasons for not being able to sleep at this age.
- An excess of *caffeine-containing drinks, alcohol* or *nicotine*, as well as *illicit drug use and withdrawal*, are additional possible influences.
- Difficulty getting off to sleep is a prominent part of adolescent *delayed sleep–wake phase disorder*). In this condition (shortly considered further in relation to excessive sleepiness as this is often the major complaint) there is a physiological inability to go to sleep until much later than the required time because of a shift in the sleep phase. The adolescent's reluctance to go to bed earlier (or the bedtime struggles of parents with younger children with this disorder) is often misinterpreted as awkward behaviour. Instead of recriminations and attempts to set limits, the timing of the sleep phase needs to be reset by means of chronotherapy (see below).

Roberts and Duong (2014) have demonstrated how sleep deprivation can cause adolescent depression which, in turn, increases the risk of decreased sleep.

Clinical scheme for the diagnosis of insomnia in children and adolescents

The correct diagnosis of the sleep disorder(s) underlying insomnia and the other sleep problems is usually achievable primarily by means of careful clinical assessment (Table 4). Polysomnography and other special investigations are rarely required.

Table 4 Clinical scheme for the diagnosis of insomnia in children and adolescents

---

General points

What is the exact nature of the problem when parents say their child does not sleep?

- What form of sleeplessness (e.g. bedtime difficulties, night walking, early morning waking) and how often the problem arises?
- A sleep diary will provide a more accurate account

Are parents' expectations reasonable?

- Do they need explanation of what is normal?
- Do they have other problems which are distorting their view?

If the child's sleep pattern is abnormal, consider the underlying sleep disorder and treat it accordingly, rather than:

- Simply reassuring parents that it is a temporary phase
- Treating it purely symptomatically with medication

Table 4 (cont.)

For this and other types of sleep problem assess the child's sleep adequately including
- A sleep history
- Review of the child's 24-hour sleep–wake pattern
- Developmental and family histories
- Review of physical and mental health

Consider general factors which may apply at any age:
- Do the parents handle the child's bedtime and general behaviour inappropriately?
- Are there other family problems that affect the child's sleeping?
- Are the sleeping circumstances unsatisfactory?
- Are there other factors preventing satisfactory sleep (i.e. poor sleep hygiene)?
- Does the child have a medical condition (including treatment) that affects sleep?

Other considerations
- The child may be of a type who generally cries more than most (including in the evening) without any organic cause
- Frequent waking and only returning to sleep by being fed suggests that the waking has been conditioned by unnecessary frequent feeding at night
- Close relationship of sleeping and other problems with certain types of food suggests allergy

Early childhood

The number and timing of daytime naps may be inappropriate.

Parental practices and the circumstances surrounding bedtime and waking during the night may be at fault.
- Is there no consistent relaxing bedtime routine?
- Is bedtime unreasonably early?
- Is bedtime and going to sleep associated with pleasant or unpleasant experiences in the child's mind?
- Does the child need his parents' presence to be able to go to sleep?
- Are the circumstances different when the child goes to sleep and when he wakes in the night?
- Do parents give in to their child's delaying tactics at bedtime or demands to be with them if he wakes during the night?
- Does the child readily settle to sleep or go back to sleep in the night with one person but not another (suggesting failure to set appropriate limits)?

Middle childhood

In addition to enquiring about the possible persistence of the above early childhood factors consider
- Over-arousal from exciting or boisterous activity near bedtime
- Night-time fears
- Worries about family or school matters which may no longer exist but have set up a habit of not sleeping well
- Being put to bed too early causing difficulty getting to sleep or waking early when sufficient sleep has been obtained for the child's age
- The child may be constitutionally unable to go to sleep until late (although other explanations should be considered first).

Table 4 (cont.)

Adolescence

Some of the above reasons for not sleeping well may still apply but the following possibilities should also be explored.

- Changes in lifestyle causing erratic sleep–wake patterns or pubertal delay in the timing of the sleep period (easily misinterpreted as 'difficult adolescent behaviour')
- Excessive intake of caffeine, alcohol, or tobacco
- Use of illegal substances
- Psychiatric disorder.

Reproduced with modifications from Stores, 2001

Excessive daytime sleepiness (hypersomnia)

Box 3 Dickens as clinical observer

Joe the Fat Boy is one of the favourite characters from the novels of Charles Dickens. He was Mr Wardle's teenage servant at Dingley Dell visited by the Pickwick Club, and was always in trouble for repeatedly falling asleep and neglecting his duties. Dickens described in clinical detail this and other aspects of Joe's behaviour including his being overweight and gluttonous as well as snoring.

Clinicians have debated the disorder of the person on whom the character of Joe might have been based, the most likely thought to be OSA. However, Joe's behaviour was sometimes bizarre and inappropriately amorous, which raises the possibility that the real person observed by Dickens might have suffered from Kleine–Levin syndrome. Additional diagnoses that have been entertained include obesity hypoventilation (Pickwickian) syndrome. The clinical picture of Joe could have been a composite of more than one sleep disorder.

Cosnett JE (1992). Charles Dickens: Observer of sleep and its disorders. *Sleep*, **15**, 264–7.

This problem has been neglected in child and adolescent psychiatry and paediatrics (Anders *et al.*, 1978), the symptoms being misperceived as laziness or lack of interest, depression or even limited intelligence. However, it has now become the subject of serious study (Kothare & Kaleyias, 2008).

- Excessive daytime sleepiness can take the form of daytime sleepiness, including actual falling asleep, or this with the addition of prolonged overnight sleep. Extreme sleepiness will cause a reduction of activity at any age, but lesser degrees in young people may produce over-activity with irritability, restlessness, poor concentration, impulsiveness or aggression leading to a diagnosis of attention deficit hyperactivity disorder without it being realized that the starting point of such behaviour was a sleep disorder rather than the reverse sequence of events (see Chapter 4).

- 'Genuine' excessive daytime sleepiness should be distinguished from fatigue or lethargy (without necessarily the need to sleep) for which different explanations are likely including physical illness. Occasionally, excessive sleepiness with long periods in bed is simulated in order to escape from a difficult situation. Detection of such cases requires careful clinical evaluation and assessment and possibly polysomnography during the sleepy periods.
- Excessive daytime sleepiness is mainly a problem in older children and especially adolescents in whom it has been associated with behavioural and psychiatric problems, as well as with educational underperformance and other risks. It is thought that many more teenagers than those who seek help are likely to be suffering from excessive sleepiness caused by chronic sleep deprivation (or 'sleep debt'). Adverse effects can be educational underperformance, road traffic accidents and other mishaps, as well as antisocial behaviour (Carskadon, 2011; Shochat *et al.*, 2014). Sometimes the situation is complicated by the use of alcohol or sedative drugs to get to sleep and/or stimulants to stay awake.

The differential diagnosis of excessive daytime sleepiness can be thought of in terms of the following three main causes.

(i) Insufficient sleep

Delayed sleep–wake *phase disorder* is a circadian rhythm disorder (Raffray *et al.*, 2011) thought to be common in adolescents, especially males. The combination of not going to sleep until late and having to get up early for school, college or work reduces the number of hours many adolescents sleep to less than that needed for satisfactory daytime functioning. The result is considerable difficulty getting up in the morning, irritability, emotional lability, and being sleepy or actually falling asleep during the day. Other complications include repeated school absences, truancy and traffic accidents.

Studies in the USA have suggested that 80% of adolescents obtain less than the average of 9 hours of sleep required for satisfactory daytime functioning (Carskadon *et al.* 2004), 25% regularly obtain less than 6 hours, and over 25% fall asleep in class. Students whose sleep becomes insufficient generally achieve lower school grades than previously (National Sleep Foundation, 2005 Sleep in America Poll). As mentioned earlier, allowing teenagers to start school lessons later in the morning is reported to improve their sleep pattern, mood and educational performance (Owens *et al.*, 2010) but there are practical difficulties in altering school day timing in this way. The 'owl' or evening chronotype is said to predispose to the delayed sleep–wake phase disorder.

The diagnostic features of delayed sleep–wake phase disorder are:

- Persistently severe difficulty getting to sleep, often until very late
- Usually uninterrupted sound sleep once it is achieved

- Considerable reluctance to get up for school, college or work. Attendance at school may be sporadic or even discontinued
- Sleepiness and underfunctioning, especially during the first part of the day, giving way to alertness in the evening and early hours
- The abnormal sleep pattern is maintained by sleeping in very late when able to do so at weekends and during holidays.

Entreaties by parents to go to sleep earlier and get up in the morning more readily are to no avail because of the changed circadian sleep–wake physiology. Treatment consists of gradually and consistently changing the sleep phase to an appropriate time. This can be achieved by slowly advancing the sleep phase (e.g. by 15 minutes a day) where the phased delay is about 3 hours or less. More severe forms of the disorder require progressive sleep phase delay in 3 hourly steps ('round the clock'). Additional measures to maintain the improved sleep schedule include early morning exposure to light and possibly the use of melatonin (Szeinberg et al., 2006). Achieving and maintaining an improved sleep–wake schedule by these means may not be easy. The difficulties are compounded if there is a vested interest in maintaining the abnormal sleep pattern, for example to avoid school ('motivated sleep phase delay'). The presence of psychological problems, including depression, may well make successful treatment less likely.

Without awareness of the delayed sleep–wake phase disorder, the condition itself can be misconstrued as 'typically difficult adolescent behaviour', laziness, school refusal, a primary depressive disorder or drug taking. Conversely, people with a psychiatric condition (including depressive illness) or neurodevelopmental disorder, such as attention deficit hyperactivity disorder or autism spectrum disorder, may have a delayed sleep phase (see Chapter 4).

- Other circadian rhythm sleep–wake disorders giving rise to both insufficient sleep and excessive daytime sleepiness were mentioned in Chapter 1. As also described in Chapter 4, advanced, irregular and non-24-hour sleep–wake rhythm disorders have been reported in some childhood neurodevelopmental disorders associated with abnormal melatonin secretion.

(ii) Disturbed nocturnal sleep

Daytime sleepiness, despite sleep duration at night being within normal limits, suggests that the restorative quality of the sleep is impaired. In childhood to adult life, poor quality sleep can be caused by the following conditions.

- *Obstructive sleep apnoea* (OSA) (Hoban & Chervin, 2007). ICSD-3 provides separate accounts of this condition in adults and children because of significant differences between them in aetiology, presentation, diagnostic criteria, course and complications.
- Paediatric OSA involves intermittent complete or partial upper airway obstruction (obstructive apnoea or hypopnoea) or both, disrupting normal ventilation during sleep. It occurs in at least 2% of children in the general population with a much higher prevalence in various childhood developmental disorders

(Grigg-Damberger & Stanley, 2011; also see sleep related breathing disorders in Chapter 3). In children in general the usual cause is enlarged tonsils and adenoids, although obesity (the main correlate in adults) is increasingly a factor and can impair the efficacy of treatment (Gozal *et al.*, 2008; Costa & Mitchell, 2009). OSA can occur at any age from the neonatal period to adolescence, although in otherwise healthy children it most commonly occurs in preschool children associated with adenotonsillar hypertrophy, and in adolescence in association with obesity.

Nighttime features suggesting OSA include loud snoring or other signs of difficulty breathing such as unusual sleeping positions, as well as restless sleep, arousals from sleep, profuse perspiration and secondary enuresis. Daytime problems can include morning headaches, excessive daytime sleepiness, and neurocognitive and behavioural problems such as antisocial behaviour, mood disorder and impaired educational performance (Gozal & Kheirandish-Gozal, 2008; Owens, 2009). Physical comorbidities can include cardiovascular problems such as pulmonary hypertension, cor pulmonale, and systemic hypertension (Teo & Mitchell, 2013), metabolic dysfunction (Gozal & Kheirandish-Gozal, 2008) and growth failure (Bonuck *et al.*, 2006).

Isolated or primary snoring (snoring unassociated with serious problems as those caused by OSA) occurs in many children and does not usually progress to OSA, and where this happens the degree of sleep apnoea tends to be mild. However, there is some evidence that primary snoring can be associated with some degree of impaired cognitive performance (Kennedy *et al.*, 2004).

In most children, treatment of OSA takes the form of adenotonsillectomy which can counter or prevent physical and psychological complications although not always (Hoban & Chervin, 2007). Other treatments are continuous positive airway pressure and weight reduction. As discussed in Chapter 4, when OSA occurs in a neurodevelopmental disorder such as Down syndrome, successful treatment may well be more difficult to achieve because of the more complicated origins of the condition compared with children in the general population.

Box 4 William Osler

Sir William Osler (1849–1919) was a Canadian physician and one time Regius Professor of Medicine at Oxford. His many outstanding contributions to medicine included detailed descriptions of clinical conditions in patients of all ages. Childhood OSA is an example:

At night the child's sleep is greatly disturbed; the respirations are loud and snoring, and there are sometimes prolonged pauses, followed by deep, noisy inspirations.

[In daytime] *The expression is dull, heavy and apathetic... In long-standing cases the child is very stupid-looking, responds slowly to questions, and may be sullen and cross.*

> **Box 4 (continued)**
>
> *Among other symptoms may be mentioned headache, which is by no means uncommon, general listlessness, and an indisposition for physical or mental exertion. The influence upon the mental development is striking.*
>
> Osler W. *The Principles and Practice of Medicine*. New York: Appleton and Co. 1892

- *Periodic limb movements in sleep* (PLMS) are periodic, highly stereotyped movements mainly of the legs occurring during sleep in both adults and children. If frequent and associated with clinically significant sleep disturbance or daytime impairment (*periodic limb movement disorder* or PLMD) (Gringras *et al.*, 2011), they can disrupt sleep and reduce its restorative properties enough to cause excessive daytime sleepiness with cognitive and behavioural change including attention deficit hyperactivity-type symptoms (Chervin *et al.*, 2002). PLMS occurs commonly in restless legs syndrome, narcolepsy, OSA and REM sleep behaviour disorder. PLMS can be associated with antidepressant medications, lithium and dopamine receptor antagonists and can be worsened by low brain iron as indicated by low serum ferritin.
- *Parasomnias* (see later in this Chapter) may disrupt sleep especially if they occur frequently. Many types are likely to be obvious but, for example, PLMS are less readily recognized clinically and require PSG or actigraphy for their detection especially those accompanied by arousals.
- *Medical and psychiatric disorders*, and some *pharmacological treatments*, can disrupt sleep, as well as *substances* such as caffeine, tobacco, alcohol and illicit drugs including their withdrawal effects.

(iii) Disorders involving an increased tendency to sleep

This occurs where excessive sleep is an intrinsic part of the condition, rather than a consequence of it.

- *Narcolepsy* (Nevsimalova, 2009), estimated to occur in about 0.1% of the United States and western European populations, is a prime example. ICSD-3 now distinguishes between narcolepsy types 1 and 2. Both types are characterized by excessive daytime sleepiness in the form of irrepressible need to sleep, including 'sleep attacks', but in type 1 this is accompanied by *cataplexy* (sudden loss of muscle tone with retention of consciousness precipitated by strong emotion). Type 1 is clearly caused by a deficiency of the neuropeptide hypocretin (orexin). Narcolepsy symptoms can be viewed as the dissociation of the component parts of REM sleep occurring separately and intruding into wakefulness. In addition to cataplexy, the classic combination consists of daytime sleep attacks, overnight sleep disruption of overnight sleep, hypnagogic and hypnopompic hallucinations, sleep paralysis and automatic behaviour, but variations in the development of these symptoms are possible.

- Cataplexy is absent in type 2 narcolepsy (which constutes the minority of narcolepsy cases) and the relationship to cerebrospinal levels of hypocretin is less definite than in type 1.
- Onset in childhood and adolescence is common but the diagnosis may not be made for several years. Reasons for this delay include misinterpretation of the symptoms as laziness or psychological disorder such as depression or conversion disorder, or they are overshadowed by the child's extreme emotional reaction to having the condition (Stores, 2006b). In young children narcolepsy can first show itself as excessively long overnight sleep or the reappearance of previously discontinued daytime napping. Narcolepsy should be considered in any young person who is excessively sleepy during the day without any obvious explanation.

Planned daytime naps, regular exercise (partly to combat excessive weight gain which is common) and medication such as modafinil can help reduce the excessive sleepiness, and cataplexy may respond to anticholinergic drugs or sodium oxybate (see Kotagal, 2012 for details). Support and advice, about education, career, and psychosocial matters, can help to improve general well-being and future prospects of children with this otherwise disabling condition.

- *Idiopathic hypersomnia* (Quinnell & Smith, 2011), seemingly rare in children, but often developing in adolescence, is generally characterized by excessive daytime sleepiness, prolonged overnight sleep and 'sleep drunkenness' (great difficulty waking in the morning or after daytime naps with confusion, disorientation, poor coordination and slowness), but none of the ancillary clinical or polysomnographic features of narcolepsy. The disorder seems to be life-long with serious psychological and social effects. Treatment is similar to that for the sleepiness of narcolepsy but may be less effective.
- *Kleine–Levin syndrome* (Arnulf et al., 2008) is rare, usually begining in the teenage years and consisting of prolonged episodes of marked hypersomnia (up to 20 hours a day) which alternate with periods of normality. When awake during episodes, patients are usually confused and in a dream-like state with anterograde amnesia. Other features can be overeating or anorexia, hypersexuality, mood change, hallucinations and delusions and other disturbed behaviours which are often bizarre and out of character. The condition is frequently mistaken for a psychological disorder or another medical condition such as cerebral tumour, encephalitis, epilepsy or substance abuse (Pike & Stores, 1994). Gradual remission usually occurs spontaneously. Both aetiology and response to treatment remain uncertain. There is some suggestion from neuroimaging and neuropsychological studies that the syndrome may not be as benign as usually considered (Miglis & Guilleminault, 2014).
- Additional causes of intermittent sleepiness in young people are *major depressive disorder, substance abuse, menstruation-related hypersomnia* and certain *other neurological diseases* including tumours within the third ventricle.

Clinical scheme for diagnosis of excessive daytime sleepiness
Table 5 gives a clinical scheme for diagnosis of excessive daytime sleepiness.

Table 5 Clinical scheme for the diagnosis of excessive daytime sleepiness

General enquiries
- Is the problem really excessive sleepiness, or fatigue or lethargy for which different explanations are likely? Check for physical illness or chronic fatigue syndrome.
- Is the complaint of sleepiness genuine or is it simulated?
- If sleepiness, how severe is it and what are its effects? (Consider behavioural effects including over-activity in young children.)
- What form of sleepiness (prolonged overnight sleep, daytime sleepiness including sleep attacks)?
- Is the sleepiness continuous or intermittent (including worse in winter)?
- Is the child on any sedating medication? Has he any neurological disorder associated with sleepiness?

At any age
Is the child getting sufficient sleep for his age (see sleep duration norms at different ages)?
- How many hours does he usually sleep?
- Does he get to sleep very late but have to get up at a certain time?
- Does he wake up by himself or have to be woken?
- Is it particularly difficult to wake him up and does he resist strongly?
Does he sleep soundly?
- Is sleep restless?
- Is it interrupted by frequent waking or other disturbance?
Is the timing of the sleep period satisfactory?
- Are daytime naps taken inappropriately for child's age?
- Is sleep divided into several periods which are irregular in their distribution or timing (irregular sleep–wake schedule)?
- Does the overnight sleep period seem to be shifted, with difficulty getting to sleep and sleeping in late when possible, e.g. weekends or holidays (delayed sleep–wake phase disorder)?
Specific features:
- Jerky legs during sleep (periodic limb movements)?
- Snoring or other noisy breathing during sleep (upper airway obstruction)? If so: apnoeic episodes or other evidence of airway obstruction during sleep?
- Other evidence of airway obstruction during sleep?
- Discrete episodes of irresistible sleep during the day? Weakness when excited or alarmed? If so, other features of narcolepsy especially hypnagogic hallucinations, sleep paralysis (narcolepsy syndrome)?
- Sleepiness despite apparently satisfactory sleep (idiopathic insomnia)?
- Recurrent periods of excessive sleepiness with normality in between? (See various causes for distinctive features.)

Table 5 (cont.)

Adolescence
Enquire about characteristic features of:
- Delayed sleep–wake phase disorder
- Other circadian rhythm sleep–wake disorders

Other considerations:
- Tobacco use, caffeine intake?
- Drugs, alcohol abuse?
- Physical illness disrupting sleep?
- Anxiety or depression?
- Other sleep disorder interfering with sleep?
- Motivated to preserve abnormal sleep pattern (school or family problems)?

Reproduced with modifications from Stores, 2001

Parasomnias and sleep related movement disorders

ICSD-3 defines parasomnias as 'abnormal sleep related complex movements, behaviours, perceptions, dreams, and autonomic nervous system activity'. Sleep related movement disorders are 'relatively simple, usually stereotyped, movements that disturb sleep or its onset' (restless legs syndrome is the exception as patients walk about or have non-stereotypical limb movements to lessen their leg discomfort). ICSD-3 follows its predecessor in having separate sections for parasomnias and sleep related movement disorders but, for present purposes, the two categories are considered together.

Many types of parasomnias and sleep related movement disorders are described in ICSD-3 many of which are seen in children and adolescents who may have more than one type. They can occur when going to sleep or waking up, during either NREM or REM sleep and sometimes inconsistently in relation to stage of sleep. The following general points about this category of sleep problems have particular implications for clinical practice. Additional details are provided elsewhere e.g. Stores (2007); Kotagal (2009).

- Precise diagnosis is important as different parasomnias may well need contrasting types of treatment. Accurate diagnosis depends principally on a detailed account of the subjective and objective sequence of events from the onset of each episode to its resolution, as well as the circumstances in which it occurs. The timing of the episodes can be important. For example, arousal disorders (such as sleepwalking or sleep terrors) usually occur in deep NREM sleep which is largely confined to the first part of the night, whereas REM-associated parasomnias, such as nightmares, occur late in sleep when that type of sleep is most prominent. Audio visual recordings combined with polysomnography can be diagnostically helpful although preliminary home audio-video recordings by parents also may reveal features omitted from usual clinical descriptions of the episodes.
- At any age, the more dramatic forms of parasomnia seem to be a main cause of diagnostic confusion and imprecision (Stores, 2010) as well as unnecessary

concern about their psychological significance as many are benign. However, parasomnias may lead to psychological complications if the child is frightened, embarrassed, or otherwise upset by the experience, or because of the reactions of other people to the episodes.

- As some childhood primary parasomnias (notably arousal disorders) tend to remit spontaneously within a few years, children and parents can often be reassured about the future, although protective measures (e.g. in severe head-banging or sleepwalking) may be required in the meantime.
- Specific treatment, including medication, is needed in only a minority of cases of primary parasomnia but is likely to be required for the underlying disorder in the secondary parasomnias. As various sleep disorders (such as OSA and periodic limb movements in sleep) can increase arousals from sleep, treatment of these co-existing disorders may help to control the occurrence of parasomnias especially arousal disorders.

Primary parasomnias

- *Hypnagogic* (sleep onset) and *hypnopompic* (on waking) *hallucination* (both benign) are common and may be frightening to the child, especially if associated with *sleep paralysis* which consists of brief inability to move or speak when falling asleep or waking up possibly with a feeling of being unable to breathe despite respiratory movements being spared. Consciousness is also preserved. The combination of sleep paralysis and hallucinosis can give rise to bizarre experiences which can be misdiagnosed as psychiatric disorder (Stores, 1998). Sleep paralysis is reported to be quite common as an isolated phenomenon but can be part of the narcolepsy syndrome.
- *Sleep related rhythmic movement disorder* (sometimes referred to as *jactatio capitis nocturna* or *jactatio corporis nocturna*) consists of repetitive, stereotyped and rhythmic movements mainly of the upper part of the body usually when going to sleep or back to sleep after waking during the night. Headbanging against a soft or hard surface is the best-known form but head rolling or rolling rocking movements of the whole body are in the same category and combinations may occur. There may be accompanying vocalizations. Some form of sleep related rhythmic movement disorder occurs in many young children, almost always remitting spontaneously by 3 to 4 years of age. When they persist, an association with attention deficit hyperactivity disorder has been reported (Stepanova *et al.*, 2005). Although alarming to parents (or a nuisance because of the noise that can be generated) they also are usually of no psychological significance unlike the persistent daytime episodes associated with severe intellectual disability. However, protective measures, such as padding the cot-sides, may be needed.
- *Arousal disorders* are a group of NREM sleep disorders the basic types of which are *sleepwalking, sleep terrors* and *confusional arousals*, all of which typically occur during the first third of the night when deep NREM sleep, from which they arise, is most prominent. The clinical features suggest a combination of being asleep and awake simultaneously. Amnesia for the episodes is partial or complete.
  - *Sleepwalking* often consists of calmly walking about in a semi-purposeful manner, mumbling or talking incoherently and acting inappropriately in

various ways. However, sleepwalking can also take an agitated form in which (as in sleep terrors) the patient appears to be very fearful and distressed, rushing about and crying out as if escaping from danger. Other complex behaviour in sleepwalking include sleep related eating disorder and, sometimes, violent or otherwise antisocial acts.

- In *sleep terrors* the child appears terrified, with staring eyes, intense sweating, rapid pulse and crying out suggesting intense distress which is apparent rather than real because he remains asleep. In both sleepwalking and sleep terrors there is a risk of accidental injury, e.g. from falling down stairs or climbing through bedroom windows.
- *Confusional arousals* occur mainly in infants and toddlers who usually remain in bed. Episodes may begin with movements and moaning before progressing to agitated and confused behaviour while they remain in bed with perhaps intense crying, calling out or thrashing about.

Arousal disorders have a strong genetic basis. They almost always resolve by adolescence or early adult life. Sleep deprivation and stress are important priming factors and episodes may be triggered, for example, by febrile illness, stress or sleep-disrupting conditions such as environmental stimuli or OSA.

Especially when the child's degree of agitation and confused behaviour is extreme, parents may well assume that he is suffering in some way. Their understandable attempts to awaken the child and comfort him should be discouraged as this may be strongly resisted and make him more agitated and confused. Instead, it is preferable to allow the behaviour to subside spontaneously while protecting the child from accidental injury. Severe forms may respond to clonazepam at bedtime. Arousal disorders can be easily confused with nocturnal seizures.

The term 'nightmare' is sometimes used inappropriately for any form of dramatic parasomnia. True *nightmares* (frightening dreams), if frequent and associated with intense bedtime fears, may indicate an anxiety disorder, and their content may suggest a cause.

- *Nocturnal enuresis* is very common. Delayed maturation often seems to be the explanation, but physical or psychological factors may be involved, especially when previous bladder control is lost. Behavioural treatment can be effective.

Secondary parasomnias

Unlike primary parasomnias, these parasomnias are manifestations of physical or psychiatric disorder.

- *Nocturnal epileptic seizures* are not uncommon in children and must be distinguished from primary parasomnias and other secondary parasomnias because of their different significance and also the investigation and treatment they require (Stores, 2013). Epilepsies in which the seizures are behavioural in type are the most likely to be misdiagnosed as non-epileptic, for example benign centro-temporal (Rolandic) epilepsy (very common in children) and nocturnal frontal lobe epilepsy, both of which are closely related to sleep.

Seizures in nocturnal frontal lobe epilepsy are particularly prone to misinterpretation as being non-epileptic. Although mainly described in adults, they also occur in children. The usual variety is often misdiagnosed mainly because of the complex motor manifestations (e.g. kicking, hitting, rocking, thrashing and cycling or scissor movements of the legs) and the accompanying vocalizations (from grunting, coughing, muttering or moaning to shouting, screaming or roaring) which characterize many attacks. These features are very different from other seizure types. The electroencephalogram may well be normal even during seizures. This and preservation of consciousness in some episodes can also suggest a non-epileptic (including an attention-seeking) basis for the attacks. The distinction between nocturnal frontal lobe epilepsy and other dramatic parasomnias, especially arousal disorders, can be difficult. Guidelines for making the distinction have been suggested (Bisulli *et al.*, 2011).

- *Other parasomnias* which are part of medical or psychiatric disorders include those associated with OSA, nocturnal asthmatic attacks or gastro-oesophageal reflux with accompanying distress, panic attacks, nocturnal disturbance that is part of post-traumatic stress disorder, and dissociative states. Symptomatic REM sleep behaviour disorder (Lloyd *et al.* 2012) in which dreams can be acted out because of a pathological preservation of muscle tone during REM sleep (likely to cause injury to oneself or others) has been reported in a number of childhood disorders (Stores, 2008). This parasomnia may be idiopathic or symptomatic of various physical disorders. Simulated parasomnias, shown by polysomnography to be enacted during wakefulness, sometimes occur in children and adolescents.

Clinical scheme for diagnosis of parasomnias
Table 6 gives a clinical scheme for diagnosis.

Table 6 Clinical scheme for the diagnosis of the parasomnias

General

A screening question for detection of parasomnias: does the child have any unusual behaviours at night such as:
- Strange sensations
- Talking, shouting, moaning or screaming
- Wandering or rushing about
- Rhythmic movements or noises
- Waking up frightened
- Wetting the bed
- Jerking of arms or legs
- Difficulty breathing
- Hurting himself.

Aspects to be considered in describing the episodes are:
- Timing (early or late in the night)
- Duration
- Physical and psychological features

Table 6 (cont.)

- Level of consciousness
- Recall or not
- Precipitating or ameliorating factors.

Precise details are needed of sequence of subjective and objective features of episodes (including timing), ideally from the start to finish, and circumstances in which they occur. Home audio-video recordings are very helpful.

Include enquiries about any daytime episodes while awake. Such episodes indicate the likelihood of a secondary parasomnia such as:

- Epilepsy
- Asthma
- Panic attacks
- Gastro-oesophageal reflux.

Consider possible combination of different attacks, each needing separate detailed assessment. Are there features possibly to suggest the parasomnias are symptomatic of underlying psychological problem? In particular:

- Frequent occurrence
- Unusually late age of onset, recurrence or persistence over many years
- Preceding trauma
- Accompanying features of psychological disorder.

Is there evidence of another sleep disorder (e.g. OSA) of which the parasomnia is one manifestation?

Specific features

Occurrence in first 2 hours of overnight sleep suggests arousal disorder characterized by

- Being inaccessible during episodes
- No recall
- Often a family history.

Occurrence late in the night suggests REM sleep related disorder especially

- True nightmares involving a frightening sequence of events (a narrative) and waking up afraid
- REM sleep behaviour disorder if behaviour during episodes reflects content of dreams.

Reproduced with modifications from Stores, 2001

References

American Academy of Sleep Medicine. *International Classification of Sleep Disorders*, 3rd edn. Darien IL: American Academy of Sleep Medicine 2014.

Anders TF, Carskadon MA, Dement WC, Harvey K. (1978). Sleep habits of children and identification of pathologically sleepy children. *Child Psychiatry Hum Dev*, **9**, 56–63.

Appleton RE, Jones AP, Gamble C *et al.* (2012). The use of melatonin in children with neurodevelopmental disorders and impaired sleep: a randomized, double-blind, placebo-controlled, parallel study (MENDS). *Health Technol Assess*, **16**, i–239.

Arnulf I, Lecendreux M, Franco P, Dauvilliers Y. (2008). Kleine–Levin syndrome: state of the art. *Rev Neurol (Paris)*, **164**, 658–68.

Bisulli F, Vignatelli L, Provini F *et al.* (2011). Parasomnias and nocturnal frontal lobe epilepsy (NFLE): lights and shadows – controversial points in the differential diagnosis. *Sleep Med*, **12** Suppl 2, S27–32.

Bjorvatin B, Pallesen S. (2009). A practical approach to circadian rhythm sleep disorders. *Sleep Med Rev*, **13**, 47–60.

Blunden S, Lushington, K, Lorenzen B *et al.* (2004). Are sleep problems under-recognised in general practice? *Arch Dis Child*, **89**, 708–12.

Bonuck K, Parikh S, Bassila M. (2006). Growth failure and sleep disordered breathing: a review of the literature. *Int J Otorhinolaryngol*, **70**, 769–78.

Brown CA, Kuo M, Phillips L, Berry R, Tan M. (2013). Non-pharmacological sleep interventions for youth with chronic health conditions: a critical review of the methodological quality of the evidence. *Disabil Rehabil*, **35**, 1221–55.

Brown RE, Basheer R, McKenna JT *et al.* (2012). Control of sleep and wakefulness. *Physiol Rev*, **92**, 1087–187.

Bruni O, Ottaviano S, Guidetti V *et al.* (1996). The Sleep Disturbance Scale for Children (SDSC). Construction and validation of an instrument to evaluate sleep disturbances in childhood and adolescence. *J Sleep Res*, **5**, 251–61.

Carskadon MA. (2011). Sleep's effects on cognition and learning in adolescence. *Prog Brain Res*, **190**, 137–43.

Carskadon MA, Acebo C, Jenni OG. (2004). Regulation of adolescent sleep: implications for behavior. *Ann NY Acad Sci*, **1021**, 276–91.

Chervin RD, Archbold KH, Dillon JE *et al.* (2002). Associations between symptoms of inattention, hyperactivity, restless legs, and periodic leg movements. *Sleep*, **25**, 213–18.

Chervin RD, Archbold KH, Panahi P, Pituch KJ. (2001). Sleep problems seldom addressed at two pediatric clinics. *Pediatrics*, **107**, 1375–80.

Chervin RD, Hedger K, Dillon JE, Pituch KJ. (2000). Pediatric sleep questionnaire (PSQ): validity and reliability of scales for sleep-disordered breathing, snoring, sleepiness, and behavioural problems. *Sleep Med*, **1**, 21–32.

Colten HR, Altevogt BM, eds. Chapter 3 Extent and health consequences of chronic sleep loss and sleep disorders; and Chapter 4 Functional and economic impact of sleep loss and sleep-related disorders. In: *Sleep Disorders and Sleep Deprivation: An Unmet Public Health Problem*. Washington DC: National Academies Press 2006. 67–209.

Costa DJ, Mitchell R. (2009). Adenotonsillectomy for obstructive sleep apnea in obese children: a meta-analysis. *Otolaryngol Head Neck Surg*, **140**, 455–60.

Crowley SJ, Acebo C, Carskadon MA. (2007). Sleep, circadian rhythms, and delayed phase in adolescence. *Sleep Med*, **8**, 602–12.

Dewald JF, Meijer AM, Oort FJ, Kerkhof GA, Bögels SM. (2010). The influence of sleep quality, sleep duration and sleepiness on school performance in children and adolescents: a meta-analytic review. *Sleep Med Rev*, **14**, 179–89.

de Weerd A, Arico I, Silvestri R. (2013). Presenting symptoms in pediatric restless legs syndrome patients. *J Clin Sleep Med*, **9**, 1077–80.

Drake C, Nickel C, Burduvali E *et al.* (2003). The Pediatric Daytime Sleepiness Scale (PDSS): sleep habits and school outcomes in middle-school children. *Sleep*, **26**, 455–8.

Ferber R. *Solve Your Child's Sleep Problems*. London: Vermilion 2013.

Fleming P, Blair P, McKenna J. (2006). New knowledge, new insights, and new recommendations. *Arch Dis Child*, **91**, 799–801.

Foster RG. (2004). Seeing the light. . . in a new way. *J Neuroendocrinol*, **16**, 179–80.

Goodlin-Jones BL, Sitnick SL, Tang K, Liu J, Anders TF. (2008). The Children's Sleep Habits Questionnaire in toddlers and preschool children. *J Dev Behav Pediatr*, **29**, 82–8.

Gozal D, Capdevila OS, Kheirandish-Gozal L. (2008). Metabolic alterations and systemic inflammation in obstructive sleep apnea among nonobese and obese prepubertal children. *Am J Respir Crit Care Med*, **177**, 1142–9.

Gozal D, Kheirandish-Gozal L. (2008). The multiple challenges of obstructive sleep apnea in children: morbidity and treatment. *Curr Opin Pediatr*, **20**, 654–8.

Gradisar M, Gardner G, Dohnt H. (2011). Recent worldwide sleep patterns and problems during adolescence: a review and meta-analysis of age, region, and sleep. *Sleep Med*, **12**, 110–18.

Gregory AM, Sadeh A. (2012). Sleep, emotional and behavioural difficulties in children and adolescents. *Sleep Med Rev*, **16**, 129–36.

Grigg-Damberger M, Stanley JJ. Sleep-related breathing disorders in children with miscellaneous neurological disorders. In: Kothare SV, Kotagal S, eds. *Sleep in Childhood Neurological Disorders*. New York; demos Medical 2011. 245–74.

Gringras JL, Gaultney JF, Picchetti DL. (2011). Pediatric periodic limb movement disorder: sleep symptom and polygraphic correlates compared with obstructive sleep apnea. *J Clin Sleep Med*, **7**, 603–9A.

Herman JH, Sheldon SH. Pharmacology of sleep disorders in children. In: Sheldon SH, Ferber R, Kryger MH, eds. *Principles and Practice of Pediatric Sleep Medicine*. Philadelphia: Elsevier Saunders 2005, 327–38.

Hoban TF, Chervin RD. Sleep-related breathing disorders of childhood: description and clinical picture, diagnosis and treatment approaches. In: Jenni OG, Carskadon MA, eds. *Sleep in Children and Adolescents* 2007, *Sleep Med Clin*, **2**, 445–62.

Hollway JA, Aman MG. (2011). Pharmacological treatment of sleep disturbance in developmental disabilities: a review of the literature. *Res Dev Disabil*, **32**, 939–62.

Jan JE, Owens JA, Weiss MD *et al.* (2008). Sleep hygiene for children with neurodevelopmental disabilities. *Pediatrics*, **122**, 1343–50.

Kennedy JD, Blunden S, Hirte C *et al.* (2004). Reduced cognition in children who snore. *Pediatr Pulmonol*, **37**, 330–7.

Kotagal S. (2009). Parasomnias in childhood. *Sleep Med Rev*, **13**, 157–68.

Kotagal S. (2012). Treatment of dyssomnias and parasomnias in childhood. *Curr Treat Options Neuro*, **14**, 630–49.

Kothare SV, Kaleyias J. (2008). Narcolepsy and other hypersomnias in children. *Curr Opin Pediatr*, **20**, 666–75.

Kuhn BR, Elliott AJ. (2003). Treatment efficacy in behavioural pediatric sleep medicine. *J Psychosom Res*, **54**, 587–97.

Kushnir J, Sadeh A. (2011). Sleep of children with night-time fears. *Sleep Med*, **12**, 870–4.

Lewandowski AS, Toliver-Sokol M, Palermo TM. (2011).Evidence-based review of subjective sleep measures. *J Pediatr Psychol*, **36**, 780–93

Lipton J, Becker RE, Kothare SV. (2008). Insomnia of childhood. *Curr Opin Pediatr*, **20**, 641–9.

Lloyd R, Tippmann-Peikert M, Sloumb N, Kotagal S. (2012). Characteristics of REM sleep behaviour disorder in childhood. *J Clin Sleep Med*, **8**, 127–31.

London New Drugs Group APC/DCT Briefing. Melatonin in paediatric sleep disorders. September 2008. *NHS National Electronic Library for Medicine website*.

Matricciani L, Blunden S, Rigney G, Williams MT, Olds TS. (2013). Children's sleep needs: is there sufficient evidence to recommend optimal sleep for children? *Sleep*, **36**, 527–34.

Meltzer LJ. (2010). Clinical management of behavioural insomnia of childhood: treatment of bedtime problems and night waking in young children. *Behav Sleep Med*, **8**, 172–89.

Meltzer LJ, Avis KT, Biggs S *et al.* (2013). The Children's Report of Sleep Patterns (CRSP): a self-report measure of sleep for school-aged children. *J Clin Sleep Med*, **9**, 235–45.

Meltzer LJ, Mindell JA. (2007). Relationship between child sleep disturbances and maternal sleep, mood, and parenting stress: a pilot study. *J Fam Psychol*, **21**, 67–73.

Meltzer LJ, Westin AM. (2011). A comparison of activity scoring rules used in pediatric research. *Sleep Med*, **12**, 793–6.

Miglis MG, Guilleminault C. (2014). Kleine–Levin syndrome: a review. *Nat Sci Sleep*, **6**, 19–26.

Mindell JA, Emslie G, Blumer J *et al.* (2006). Pharmacological management of insomnia in children and adolescents: consensus statement. *Pediatrics*, **117**, e1223–32.

Mirmiran M, Maas YG, Ariagno RL. (2003). Development of fetal and neonatal sleep and circadian rhythms. *Sleep Med Rev*, **7**, 321–4.

Morrell JM. (1999). The role of maternal cognitions in infant sleep problems as assessed by a new instrument, the maternal cognitions about infant sleep questionnaire. *J Child Psychol Psychiatry*, **40**, 247–58.

National Sleep Foundation. *Sleep in America Poll 2005*. Washington DC: National Sleep Foundation 2006.

Nevsimalova S. (2009). Narcolepsy in childhood. *Sleep Med Rev*. **13**, 169–80.

Owens JA. (2008). Classification and epidemiology of childhood sleep disorders. *Prim Care*, **35**, 533–46.

Owens JA. (2009). Neurocognitive and behavioural impact of sleep disordered breathing in children. *Pediatr Pulmonol*, **44**, 417–22.

Owens JA, Babcock D, Blumer J *et al.* (2005). The use of pharmacotherapy in the treatment of pediatric insomnia in primary care: rational approaches. A consensus meeting summary. *J Clin Sleep Med*, **1**, 49–59.

Owens JA, Belon K, Moss P. (2010). Impact of delaying school start time on adolescent sleep, mood, and behaviour. *Arch Pediatr Adolesc Med*, **164**, 608–14.

Owens JA, Dalzell V. (2005). Use of the BEARS sleep screening tool in a pediatric residents' continuity clinic: a pilot study. *Sleep Med*, **6**, 63–9.

Owens JA, Moturi S. (2009). Pharmacological treatment of pediatric insomnia. *Child Adolesc Psychiatr Clin N Am*, **18**, 1001–16.

Owens JA, Spirito A, McGuinn M. (2000). The Children's Sleep Habits Questionnaire (CSHQ): psychometric properties of a survey instrument for school-aged children. *Sleep*, **23**, 1043–51.

Pelayo R, Dubic M. (2008). Pediatric sleep pharmacology. *Semin Pediatr Neurol*, **15**, 79–90.

Pike M, Stores G. (1994). Kleine–Levin syndrome: a cause of diagnostic confusion. *Arch Dis Child*, **71**, 355–7.

Pressman MR. (2007). Factors that predispose, prime and precipitate NREM parasomnias in adults: clinical and forensic implications. *Sleep Med Rev*, **11**, 5–30.

Quine L. *Solving Children's Sleep Problems: A Step by Step Guide for Parents*. Huntingdon: Beckett Karlson 1997.

Quinnell TG, Smith IE. (2011). Narcolepsy, idiopathic hypersomnolence and related conditions. *Clin Med*, **11**, 282–6.

Raffray T, Van Reen E, Tarokh L, Carskadon MA. Circadian rhythm disorders. In: Kothare SV, Kotagal S, eds. *Sleep in Childhood Neurological Disorders*. New York: demos Medical 2011. 219–233.

Roberts RE, Duong HT. (2014). The prospective association between sleep deprivation and depression among adolescents. *Sleep*, **37**, 239–44.

Robinson AM, Richdale AL. (2004). Sleep problems in children with an intellectual disability: parental perceptions of sleep problems, and views of treatment effectiveness. *Child Care Health Dev*, **30**, 139–50.

Sadeh A, Tikotsky L, Scher A. (2010). Parenting and infant sleep. *Sleep Med Rev*, **14**, 89–96.

Schnoes CJ, Kuhn BR, Workman EF, Ellis CR. (2006). Pediatric prescribing practices for clonidine and other pharmacological agents for children with sleep disturbance. *Clin Pediatr (Phila)*, **45**, 229–38.

Shochat T, Cohen-Zion M, Tzischinsky O. (2014). Functional significance of inadequate sleep in adolescents: A systematic review. *Sleep Med Rev*, **18**, 75–87.

Simakajornboon N, Kheirandish-Gozal L, Gozal D. (2009). Diagnosis and management of restless legs syndrome in children. *Sleep Med Rev*, **13**, 149–56.

Simonds JF, Parraga H. (1982). Prevalence of sleep disorders and sleep behaviors in children and adolescents. *J Am Acad Child Psychiatry*, **21**, 383–8.

Smaldone A, Honig JC, Byrne MW. (2007). Sleepless in America; inadequate sleep and relationships to health and well-being of our nation's children. *Pediatrics*, **119** Suppl 1, S29–37.

Spruyt K, Gozal D. (2011). Pediatric sleep questionnaires as diagnostic and epidemiological tools: a review of currently available instruments. *Sleep Med Rev*, **15**, 19–32.

Spruyt K, Molfese DL, Gozal D. (2011). Sleep duration, sleep regularity, body weight, and metabolic homeostasis in school-aged children. *Pediatrics*, **127**, e345–52.

Stepanova I, Nevsimilova S, Hanusova J. (2005). Rhythmic movement disorder in sleep persisting into childhood and adulthood. *Sleep*, **28**, 851–7.

St James-Roberts I. (2008). Infant crying and sleeping: helping parents to prevent and manage problems. *Prim Care*, **35**, 547–67.

Stores G. (1998). Sleep paralysis and hallucinosis. *Behav Neurol*, **11**, 109–12.

Stores G. *A Clinical Guide to Sleep Disorders in Children and Adolescents*. Cambridge: Cambridge University Press 2001.

Stores G. (2006a). Sleep disorders. In: Gillberg C, Harrington R, Steinhausen H-C, eds. *A Clinician's Handbook of Child and Adolescent Psychiatry*. Cambridge: Cambridge University Press 2006. 304–38.

Stores G. (2006b). The protean manifestations of childhood narcolepsy and their misinterpretation. *Dev Med Child Neurol*, **48**, 307–10.

Stores G. (2007). Parasomnias of childhood and adolescence. *Sleep Med Clin*, **2**, 405–17.

Stores G. (2008). Rapid eye movement sleep behaviour disorder in children and adolescents. *Dev Med Child Neurol*, **50**, 728–32.

Stores G. (2010). Dramatic parasomnias: recognition and treatment. *Br J Hosp Med*, **71**, 505–10.

Stores G. (2013). Sleep disturbance in childhood epilepsy: clinical implications, assessment and treatment. *Arch Dis Child*, **98**, 548–51.

Szeinberg A Borodkin K, Dagan Y. (2006). Melatonin treatment in adolescents with delayed sleep phase syndrome. *Clin Pediatr (Phila)*, **45**, 809–18.

Teo DT, Mitchell RB. (2013). Systematic review of effect of adenotonsillectomy on cardiovascular parameters in children with obstructive sleep apnea. *Otolaryngol Head Neck Surg*, **148**, 21–8.

Tietze AL, Blankenburg M, Hechler T *et al.* (2012). Sleep disturbance in children with multiple disabilities. *Sleep Med Rev*, **16**, 117–27.

Werner H, LeBourgeois MK, Geiger A, Jenni OG. (2009). Assessment of chronotype in four- to eleven-year-old children: reliability and validity of the children's chronotype questionnaire (CCTQ). *Chronobiol Int*, **26**, 992–1014.

Wiggs L. (2009). Behavioural aspects of children's sleep. *Arch Dis Child*, **94**, 59–62.

Wolfson AR, Carskadon MA. (2003). Understanding adolescents' sleep patterns and school performance: a critical appraisal. *Sleep Med Rev*, **7**, 491–506.

2

Special considerations regarding sleep disturbance in children with a neurodevelopmental disorder

The general content of the last chapter is directly relevant to consideration of sleep disturbance in children with a neurodevelopmental disorder, but the following supplementary points need to be made in this chapter concerning this particular group of children.

Sleep is a relatively neglected aspect of childhood neurodevelopmental disorders

It was claimed at the start of this book that there are serious shortcomings regarding sleep and its disorders in the education of both the general public (including parents) and also in the training of physicians and other child healthcare professionals. One consequence is that research on childhood sleep issues has been limited, notably in the field of neurodevelopmental disorders where sleep problems loom particularly large. Relatively few studies have achieved the highest methodological standards. Shortcomings have included small sample sizes, lack of randomized controlled research design, possible recruitment bias, inadequate assessment of specific sleep disorders underlying the children's sleep problems, and also the effects of treatments. In addition, aetiological factors capable of contributing to sleep disturbance, including comorbidities, have not always been considered. Not surprisingly, findings do not always agree or provide adequate insights. That said, the literature, as it stands, can still suggest important possibilities which can act as a guide to diagnostic assessment and treatment approaches for use in clinical practice.

General points

When individual neurodevelopmental disorders are reviewed in Chapter 4, it will be evident that certain points need to be repeated from one condition to another. It follows from what has just been said that one of them is the need for further well-designed research. Others are the multifactorial aetiology of the sleep disturbance (with its implications for the assessment and treatment programmes required), and the usual need for multidisciplinary investigation and care involving help, advice and support for parents and other carers. Long-term surveillance will usually be required, and treatment might need to be revised as family circumstances and attitudes affecting sleep may have changed.

Children with neurodevelopmental disorders do not have a separate set of sleep disorders

Although different polysomnographic phenotypes have been described in some neurodevelopmental disorders (Harvey & Kennedy, 2002), from the clinical point of view, children with neurodevelopmental problems basically have the same range of sleep disorders as other children (see Chapter 1). However, their problems are generally more prevalent and severe and, if untreated, more persistent. Also, because of the likely multifactorial aetiology of their sleep disturbance, assessment and treatment might well have to be more complicated than in other children. The psychological, social and other adverse effects of the neurodevelopmental disorder itself may be worsened by the sleep disturbance.

The aetiology of sleep disturbance in children with a neurodevelopmental disorder is usually multifactorial

In addition to the aetiological factors that may operate in any child's sleep disturbance, there may be additional considerations concerning children whose development is compromised. Such factors are considered in the accounts in Chapter 4 of individual neurodevelopmental disorders.

If a child has an *intellectual disability* or *communication problems*, his ability to learn good sleep habits may be impaired. For example, understanding of requests may be limited and so might awareness of environmental time cues. *Intrinsic factors* may operate to disturb sleep. For instance, a melatonin abnormality has been described in autism and Smith–Magenis syndrome affecting sleep–wake patterns, possibly contributing to both insomnia and daytime sleepiness problems and their behavioural consequences. *Medical and psychiatric comorbidities* capable of contributing to sleep disturbance feature prominently in the neurodevelopmental disorders. Main examples are considered in the next chapter. Possible *medication effects* were discussed in Chapter 1.

Parenting factors can be particularly prominent. Possibly because of over-concern about their child's welfare and safety, parents of children with a developmental disorder may inadvertently reinforce their child's problem behaviour at bedtime or during the night by paying attention to him for long periods or having him share their bed. They may have special difficulty with implementing sleep hygiene principles or complying with behavioural treatment procedures. Their difficulties are likely to be increased if they are stressed (Byars *et al.*, 2011), if they themselves are sleep deprived, anxious and depressed because of their child's sleep problem (Meltzer & Mindell, 2007), and if their knowledge about children's sleep is inadequate, as may well be the case without informed help and advice. Such problems are likely to be intensified if their child has any chronic condition (Melzer & Moore, 2008; Hysing *et al.*, 2009). Because of the various pressures of bringing up a child with a development delay, parents' mental health and relationships are likely to suffer, further affecting their ability to cope (Quine, 1992).

Such aetiological complexity is a major theme regarding assessment and treatment both of which will need to be more comprehensive than is usual in typically developing children with a sleep disturbance. Adequate investigation and management may seem like a daunting task and may well require specialist help, but there is no alternative to this detailed approach because of the essentially complicated nature of the problem.

Sleep assessments should be basically the same as for other children but with some modifications

In principle, the same assessment procedure outlined in Chapter 1 for the investigation of sleep disturbance in children in general can be followed for those with a neurodevelopmental disorder. However, some additional considerations are appropriate.

As disturbed sleep might be given inadequate attention among the various other aspects of the child's condition and the family's predicament, routine screening for sleep problems should be considered mandatory, followed by diagnosis of the sleep disorder(s) underlying any sleep problem identified in this way. Follow-up and repeated screening for sleep disturbance and possible emergence of aetiological factors following initial assessment should form part of continuing care. Screening may be best undertaken, and subsequent action initiated and coordinated, by the lead paediatric team especially if the child requires attendance at a variety of specialized paediatric services.

For usual clinical purposes, parents are the main informants but children themselves might be able to contribute, although this may well be limited by their intellectual limitations or communication problems. Parents may be all too aware of their child's insomnia problems but excessive sleepiness can be viewed as less problematic or even a respite from difficult behaviour or their other problems. In theory, accurate assessment of parasomnias can rely heavily on subjective information from the patient. However, in many cases parents' observations or video recordings have to suffice. The Children's Sleep Habits Questionnaire was mentioned in Chapter 1 as a possibly useful adjunct to history-taking questions as a screening measure for children in general. The Modified Simonds and Parraga Sleep Questionnaire, which has been used, for example, in children with autistic spectrum disorders (Johnson *et al.* 2012), is a suitable alternative.

For the diagnosis of certain sleep disorders (e.g. OSA or sleep–wake cycle disorders), objective confirmation and clarification of parental reports of symptoms of a sleep problem should be obtained. However, compliance with objective sleep assessments (actometry or polysomnography) can be difficult to achieve depending on a child's ability to understand and accept the procedure. Such difficulties can be overestimated and their risk reduced by staff experienced with neurodevelopmentally disabled children and with their parents closely involved in the procedures (Paasch *et al.*, 2012).

With some modifications basic treatment principles apply as in other children

As in any patient, appropriate advice and choice of treatment from the many types now possible depends essentially on the nature of a child's sleep disorder. It is worth re-emphasizing that treatment of a sleep disturbance should not precede diagnosis of the underlying cause. Although in most other forms of medical practice the distinction between a health problem or complaint and its underlying cause is axiomatic, this distinction does not always apply in the case of sleep disturbance. As a result, the cause of the sleep disturbance may not be identified and attempts made to treat the problem symptomatically may well prove unsuccessful. However, efficacy may be different in the presence of a neurodevelopmental disorder if only because of possible compliance problems, although this can be often over-emphasized.

Because of the usually complex aetiology and the potential chronicity of sleep disturbances in children with a neurodevelopmental disorder, treatment programmes of any type are likely also to require a skilled, experienced and multidisciplinary approach. However, the prospect of successful treatment can easily be under-estimated with failure to adopt appropriate, forward-looking strategies (Grigg-Damberger & Ralls (2013). That said, as discussed in Chapter 1, a positive approach to treatment possibilities has to be tempered by acknowledging that more sophisticated research is required concerning the efficacy of sleep treatments, perhaps especially in the case of children with neurodevelopmental disorders. Research on non-pharmacological treatments for sleep disturbances in children with neurodevelopmental disorders and other chronic conditions, such as intellectual disability or visual impairment, was considered by Brown *et al.* (2013) to be methodologically weak. However, the authors added the rider that some interventions, including those of a behavioural nature, were promising and appropriate to use with some expectation that they might be effective.

It can be seen from the review of behavioural approaches by Richdale and Wiggs (2005), and that by Hollway and Aman (2011) concerning pharmacological treatments, that the sleep disorders of developmentally disabled children may be as treatable as in other children. If parents are disabused of the idea that serious sleep problems (and their consequences for the child and also their own well-being) are inevitable, the uptake of the available treatments, which can be poor (Wiggs & Stores, 1996), would be improved. However, this would require a corresponding increased awareness by professionals of the various treatment possibilities.

It might be assumed that behavioural methods of treatment are likely to be less successful in children with neurodevelopmental disorders compared with other children. Richdale and Wiggs (2005) discuss evidence to the contrary. They argue that such methods have the advantages that they utilize non-verbal means of modifying behaviour, can be individually designed to suit the particular needs and circumstances of each child and also his family who may be faced with complex and multiple problems, and, if successful, may improve the child's behaviour and also parental well-being.

Based on their review of the increasing number of studies of behavioural treatment of insomnia in children with various types of developmental disorder, these authors conclude that, despite the mixed nature of the studies they analysed (including the range of methodological sophistication), insomnia in children with developmental delay can be usefully treated by means of various behavioural methods. Extinction and graduated extinction methods most merited the accolade of being 'probably efficacious'. Other methods were felt to need further evaluation. Preliminary findings suggest that behavioural treatment for insomnia problems in the form of booklet instruction for parents can be as effective as face-to-face contact with a therapist (Montgomery *et al.*, 2004).

In the same review, Richdale and Wiggs (2005) went on to consider the possible value of behavioural treatments for sleep–wake rhythm disorders and some parasomnias (sleep terrors and rhythmic movement disorders such as headbanging). Their overall conclusion this time was that studies are either non-existent or so limited that they can only be called experimental. The authors' parting shots were that, especially for 'hard to treat' children, combinations of behavioural and pharmacological treatments need to be explored; and (obviously) there is a need for quality research in the field of children's sleep disorders generally, but especially concerning children with a developmental disorder.

As mentioned in Chapter 1, pharmacological treatment has a limited part to play in the treatment of children's sleep disorders. That said, it is felt that medications for otherwise treatment-resistant paediatric insomnia might well (with further evidence) be justified, especially in children with neurodevelopmental disorders, chronic medical conditions and psychiatric disorders (Owens *et al.*, 2005; Mindell *et al.*, 2006). Combinations of behavioural and pharmacological treatments might be required although not yet adequately studied.

Hollway and Aman (2011) conducted a comprehensive literature search concerning the pharmacological treatment of insomnia in patients with a developmental disability, mainly children and adolescents. The range of medications covered by this review was wide, comprising antihistamines, melatonin and melatonin agonists, alpha-adrenergic agonists/anti-adrenergics, benzodiazepines, non-benzodiazepine, GABAergic (z) drugs, cyclic antidepressants, atypical antipsychotics and conventional antipsychotics. Trazodone, mirtazepine and ramelteon were considered promising by the reviewers. Despite its frequent use for children in general, diphenhydramine was considered to lack empirical evidence of effectiveness, clonidine had not been adequately studied, zolpidem has been shown to be ineffective, and the use of benzodiazepines and imipramine was considered to be hampered by the risk of side-effects.

Attention to family including parenting issues is essential

Particular attention needs to be paid to the emotional state of parents of children with a neurodevelopmental disorder. The effects on child development of persistently disturbed sleep, including family effects, were discussed in Chapter 1. These issues can be especially important for assessment and treatment in the case of children with a neurodevelopmental disorder whose parents are frequently faced with considerable concerns and challenges. For example, such parents often find coping with the disturbed behaviours (including psychiatric disorders) more difficult than dealing with other aspects of the disorder. As these problems may be caused or worsened by the child's sleep disturbance, it is important that the cause of the sleep problem is ascertained and treated effectively as far as possible.

Some mothers of children with an intellectual disability and severe sleep problem have been described as more irritable, concerned about their own health and less affectionate towards their children (with greater use of physical punishment) than mothers of such children without sleep problems as reported by Quine (1992). There have been suggestions that marital discord and separation, and even physical abuse of children, may result (Chavin & Tinson, 1980).

A number of other studies have been concerned with the inter-relationships between sleep disturbance in children with developmental disorders and their parents' own sleep quality. Chu and Richdale (2009) reported how children's sleep and behaviour problems were associated with disturbed sleep and increased depression, anxiety and stress levels in their mothers, whose own sleep disturbance was predictive of their psychological well-being. Gallagher et al. (2010) also emphasized stress as being associated with poor sleep quality in parents caring for children with developmental disabilities. Obviously, it is important to identify families in which such complications are likely to occur, and to intervene at an early stage. Psychosocial disadvantage and parental psychiatric disorder are likely warning signs. There have been indications that treatment of her children's sleep problems can improve a mother's mental state, confidence in her own parenting ability and her relationships with her child, and also her child's behaviour (Wolfson et al., 1992; Quine, 1992; Minde et al., 1994; Wiggs & Stores, 1998). Beneficial effects may be greater in mothers than in fathers (Wiggs & Stores, 2001).

Risk of misinterpretation and misdiagnosis of sleep disorders

This risk exists in all subjects of whatever age (Stores, 2010) but may be increased in children with developmental disorders in whom unusual behaviours can be wrongly attributed to their basic condition rather than being recognized as features of a sleep disorder. Failure to recognize that the starting point of any child's psychological problems has, in fact, been a sleep disorder readily leads to inappropriate referral to educational or psychiatric services alone. The possibility that disturbed sleep might lie behind or contribute to the child's psychological difficulties should be considered (alongside other more conventionally acknowledged influences) with appropriate enquiries about the child's sleep. This requires more attention being paid to sleep history-taking than is usual in clinical practice (Owens, 2001).

The approach and attention to detail required in correctly recognizing sleep disturbance by means of screening, avoiding its misdiagnosis as some other condition, and identifying the precise underlying sleep disorder on which a correct choice of treatment can be based, are amply justified in view of the benefits to the child with a neurodevelopmental disorder and his family that should accrue. His basic condition may not be alterable but, in principle, attention to his sleep disturbance can be expected to improve his developmental status and general circumstances, with better prospects in adult life.

The need to be mindful of cultural issues (discussed in the introduction of this book) applies to possible cultural differences in the interpretation of sleep phenomena as abnormal or not.

Brown CA, Kuo M, Phillips L, Berry R, Tan M. (2013). Non-pharmacological sleep interventions for youth with chronic health conditions: a critical review of the methodological quality of the evidence. *Disabil Rehabil*, **35**, 1221–55.

Byars KC, Yeomans-Maldonado G, Noll JG. (2011). Parental functioning and pediatric sleep disturbance: an examination of factors associated with parenting stress in children clinically referred for evaluation of insomnia. *Sleep Med*, **12**, 898–905.

Chavin W, Tinson S. (1980). The developing child: children with sleep difficulties. *Health Visit*, **53**, 477–80.

Chu J, Richdale AL. (2009). Sleep quality and psychological wellbeing in mothers of children with developmental disabilities. *Res Dev Disabil*, **30**, 1512–22.

Gallagher S, Phillips AC, Carroll D. (2010). Parental stress is associated with poor sleep quality in parents caring for children with developmental disabilities. *J Pediatr Psychol*. **35**, 728–37.

Grigg-Damberger M, Ralls F. (2013). Treatment strategies for complex behavioural insomnia in children with neurodevelopmental disorders. *Curr Opin Pulm Med*, **19**, 616–25.

Harvey MT, Kennedy CH. (2002). Polysomnographic phenotypes in developmental disabilities. *Int J Devl Neuroscience*, **20**, 443–8.

Hollway JA, Aman MG. (2011). Pharmacological treatment of sleep disturbance in developmental disabilities: a review of the literature. *Res Dev Disabil*, **32**, 939–62.

Hysing M, Sivertsen B, Stormark KM, Elgen I, Lundervold AJ. (2009). Sleep in children with chronic illness, and the relation to emotional and behavioural problems – a population-based study. *J Pediatr Psychol*, **34**, 665–70.

Johnson CR, Turner KS, Foldes EL, Malow BA, Wiggs L. (2012). Comparison of sleep questionnaires in the assessment of sleep disturbances in children with autism spectrum disorders. *Sleep Med*, **13**, 795–801.

Meltzer LJ, Mindell JA. (2007). Relationship between child sleep disturbances and maternal sleep, mood, and parenting stress: a pilot study. *J Fam Psychol*, **21**, 67–73.

Meltzer LJ, Moore M. (2008). Sleep disruptions in parents of children and adolescents with chronic illnesses: prevalence, causes, and consequences. *J Pediatr Psychol*, **33**, 279–91.

Minde K, Faucon A, Falkner S. (1994). Sleep problems in toddlers: effects of treatment on their daytime behaviour. *J Am Acad Child Adolesc Psychiatry*, **33**, 1114–21.

Mindell JA, Emslie G, Blumer J *et al.* (2006). Pharmacological management of insomnia in children and adolescents: consensus statement. *Pediatrics*, **117**, e1223–32.

Montgomery P, Stores G, Wiggs L. (2004). The relative efficacy of two brief treatments for sleep problems in young learning disabled (mentally retarded) children: a randomised controlled trial. *Arch Dis Child*, **89**, 125–130.

Owens JA. (2001). The practice of pediatric sleep medicine: results of a community survey. *Pediatrics*, **108**, E51.

Owens JA, Babcock D, Blumer J *et al.* (2005). The use of pharmacotherapy in the treatment of pediatric insomnia in primary care: rational approaches. A consensus meeting summary. *J Clin Sleep Med*, **1**, 49–59.

Paasch V, Hoosier TM, Accardo J, Ewen JB, Slifer KJ. (2012). Technical tips: performing EEGs and polysomnograms on children with neurodevelopmental disabilities. *Neurodiagn J*, **52**, 333–48.

Quine L. (1992). Severity of sleep problems in children with severe learning difficulties: description and correlates. *J Community Appl Soc*, **2**, 247–68.

Richdale A, Wiggs L (2005). Behavioral approaches to the treatment of sleep problems in children with developmental disorders: What is the state of the art? *Int J Behav Consult Ther*, **1**, 165–89.

Stores G. Misdiagnosis of sleep disorders in adults and children. In: Cappuccio FP, Miller MA, Lockley SW, eds. *Sleep, Health, and Society from Aetiology to Public Health*. Oxford: Oxford University Press 2010 300–24.

Wiggs L, Stores G. (1996). Sleep problems in children with severe intellectual disabilities: What help is being provided? *J Appl Res Intellect*, **9**, 159–64.

Wiggs L, Stores G. (1998). Behavioural treatment for sleep problems in children with severe intellectual disabilities and daytime challenging behaviour: effects on sleep patterns of mother and child. *J Sleep Res*, **7**, 119–26.

Wiggs L, Stores G. (2001). Behavioural treatment for sleep problems in children with severe intellectual disabilities and daytime challenging behaviour: effect on mothers and fathers. *Br J Health Psychol*, **6** (pt 3), 257–69.

Wolfson A, Lacks P, Futterman A. (1992). Effect of parent training on infant sleep patterns, parent stress, and perceived parental competence. *J Consult Clin Psychol*, **60**, 41–8.

3

Main comorbid conditions in neurodevelopmental disorders capable of contributing to sleep disturbance

Because it is so common in neurodevelopmental disorders, comorbidity is a particularly important issue in the overall care of children with such disorders including attention to their sleep disturbance. The term 'comorbidity' has been defined in various ways by different authors (Bax & Gillberg, 2010) and there is no overall agreement about what it should imply. For present purposes, the term is used to mean simply the co-occurrence of disorders more frequently than would be expected by chance. It will also refer to some conditions themselves capable of disturbing sleep, whether they are usually viewed as coexisting with a neurodevelopmental disorder or considered to be part of its accepted phenotype.

To achieve insight into the reasons for the sleep disturbance in the individual child, it is necessary to identify any such comorbid conditions and to know in what way they may be contributing to his sleep problem. Attention to these comorbidities (as far as possible) will be necessary to achieve optimum improvement in the child's sleep and overall well-being, as well as that of his family. Attention to comorbidity issues can mean complex assessment and management procedures which, however, are necessary to gain adequate insight into the individual child's sleep disturbance and to indicate overall treatment requirements.

In the neurodevelopmental disorders there are many possible conditions which can be comorbid. In this chapter, attention is confined to main comorbidities described in the Chapter 4 accounts of specific neurodevelopmental disorders for which there is evidence that sleep disturbance can be a significant feature. Only some aspects of connections between each comorbidity and sleep are mentioned. More general accounts of medical and psychiatric comorbidities affecting sleep have been provided by Stores and Wiggs (2001), Bandla and Splaingard (2004), and Palermo and Owens (2008).

In addition to the following comorbidities, as indicated in the Chapter 4 account of each neurodevelopmental disorder, one or more other neurodevelopmental disorders may be comorbid with the one in question.

Bandla H, Splaingard M. (2004). Sleep problems in children with common medical disorders. *Pediatr Clin North Am*, **51**, 203–27.

Bax M, Gillberg C., eds. *Comorbidities in Developmental Disorders*. Clinics in Developmental Medicine No. 187. London: Mac Keith Press 2010.

Palermo TM, Owens J. (2008). Introduction to the special issue: sleep in pediatric medical populations. *J Pediatr Psychol*, **33**, 227–31.

Stores G, Wiggs L., eds. *Sleep Disturbance in Children and Adolescents with Disorders of Development: its Significance and Management.* Clinics in Developmental Medicine No. 155. London: Mac Keith Press 2001.

Intellectual disability

Neurodevelopment disorders often include intellectual impairment to varying degrees. Early reports about severely intellectually impaired children all demonstrated high rates of serious and persistent sleep problems, often associated with disturbed behaviour and family difficulties (Stores, 1992). Later reports, for example by Didden *et al.* (2002), Robinson and Richdale (2004), Dorris *et al.* (2008), Lipton *et al.* (2008), and Chu and Richdale (2009), have confirmed this link between intellectual disability and sleep disturbance.

Intellectual impairment can lead to sleep disturbance in various ways, including as a result of damage to sleep mechanisms and systems, and to differing extents.

As mentioned earlier, from birth through infancy, the biological clock controlling sleep and wakefulness has to develop in response to perception of environmental indicators of time ('zeitgebers'). This process by which the circadian rhythm is established includes appreciation of the 24 hour light–dark cycle and timing of meals and social contacts. Awareness of these indicators may be impaired by maldevelopment of or damage to the anatomical and neurotransmitter systems in the brain involved in the control of sleep and wakefulness described by Brown *et al.* (2012).

Extensive and severe brain damage produces an 'acerebrate' state in which there is little response to external stimuli and often a highly irregular sleep–wake pattern (Okawa & Sasaki, 1987). In this state, as normal sleep phenomena (such as sleep spindles and vertex sharp waves) are usually lacking, it is difficult to distinguish between sleeping and the awake state ('monostage sleep'). Children who are less severely damaged, but whose perception and social awareness are severely impaired, may not entrain their sleep–wake rhythms to a 24 hour period and therefore exhibit a 'free-running' circadian rhythm which is not synchronized to zeitgebers, describing an endogenous rhythm of about 25 hours.

Polysomnographic studies have for long been concerned with the relationship between intellectual level and REM sleep. As the proportion of this type of sleep is high in neonates, decreasing as the infant matures, it might be expected that children with a neurodevelopmental disorder would have an immature pattern of brain activity with more REM sleep than typically developing children. In fact, they were reported to have less. These findings support the view that REM sleep is somehow involved in the learning process (Siegel, 2001). Intellectual disability has also been linked with abnormalities of sleep spindle activity which has been associated with the memorizing process (Tamminen *et al.*, 2010).

Interesting though such reports may be, studies of mixed groups of developmentally delayed children have the disadvantage of involving generalizations across a wide variety of different conditions. A more discriminating approach has examined relationships between intellectual disability and sleep by exploring possible polysomnographic phenotypes analogous to behavioural phenotypes in specific developmental disability syndromes as described by O'Brien (2011).

Harvey and Kennedy (2002) reviewed the relatively few studies of this type and concluded that differences in sleep architecture appear to be discernible between autism, Down syndrome and fragile X syndrome. In keeping with earlier studies of patients with intellectual disabilities in general, REM sleep abnormalities (including a deficiency) are more common in all groups compared with normal controls. Studies in children with Angelman syndrome have also demonstrated REM sleep deficiency (Miano *et al.* 2004). However, the feature of more specific clinical value in this syndrome is the occurrence of various types of rhythmic slow activity sometimes with spikes or sharp waves (Vendrame *et al.*, 2012) which, although not diagnostic, can be suggestive of this syndrome at an early age. Miano *et al.* (2008) have reported sleep microstructure differences between Down syndrome and fragile X syndrome. How far these physiological differences relate to clinical sleep disorders has yet to be determined.

The high rates of sleep disturbance (which almost invariably mainly involves insomnia) associated with intellectual disability can be accounted for by other factors additional to intrinsic factors such as those just discussed. These include commonly co-occurring psychiatric disorders (especially autism spectrum disorder, attention deficit hyperactivity disorder and conduct disorders) (Einfeld *et al.*, 2011), and the harmful effects on parenting abilities that can occur (Quine, 1992). Despite the consistent evidence of the commonness and serious consequences of sleep disturbance in children with an intellectual disability, the impression gained is that the shortcomings in the help given to such children and their families to which attention was drawn some time ago (Wiggs & Stores, 1996) can still persist (MacCrosain & Byrne, 2009).

Brown RE, Basheer R, McKenna JT, Strecker RE, McCarley RW. (2012). Control of sleep and wakefulness. *Physiol Rev*, **92**, 1087–187.

Chu J, Richdale AL. (2009). Sleep quality and psychological wellbeing in mothers of children with developmental disabilities. *Res Dev Disabil*, **30**, 1512–22.

Didden R, Korzilius H, van Aperlo B, van Overloop C, de Vries M. (2002). Sleep problems and daytime problem behaviours in children with intellectual disability. *J Intellect Disabil Res*, **46** (Pt 2), 537–47.

Dorris L, Scott N, Zuberi S, Gibson N, Espie C. (2008). Sleep problems in children with neurological disorders. *Dev Neurorehabil*, **11**, 95–114.

Einfeld SL, Ellis LA, Emerson E. (2011). Comorbidity of intellectual disability and mental disorder in children and adolescents: a systematic review. *J Intellect Dev Disabil*, **36**, 137–43.

Harvey MT, Kennedy CH (2002). Polysomnographic phenotypes in developmental disabilities. *Int J Devl Neuroscience*, **20**, 443–8.

Lipton J, Becker RE, Kothare SV. (2008). Insomnia of childhood. *Curr Opin Pediatr*, **20**, 641–9.

MacCrosain AM, Byrne MC. (2009). Are we ignoring the problem of sleep disorder in children with intellectual disabilities? *Ir J Med Sci*, **178**, 427–31.

Miano S, Bruni O, Elia M *et al.* (2008). Sleep phenotypes of intellectual disability: a polysomnographic evaluation in subjects with Down syndrome, and fragile-X syndrome. *Clin Neurophysiol*, **119**, 1242–7.

Miano S, Bruni O, Leuzzi V *et al.* (2004). Sleep polygraphy in Angelman syndrome. *Clin Neurophysiol*, **115**, 938–45.

O'Brien G. *Behavioural Phenotypes*. Cambridge: Cambridge University Press 2011.

Okawa M, Sasaki H. Sleep disorders in mentally retarded and brain-impaired children. In: Guilleminault C., ed. *Sleep and its Disorders in Children*. New York: Raven Press 1987 269–90.

Quine L. (1992). Severity of sleep problems in children with severe learning difficulties: description and correlates. *J Community Appl Soc*, **2**, 247–68.

Robinson AM, Richdale AL. (2004). Sleep problems in children with an intellectual disability: parental perceptions of sleep problems, and views of treatment effectiveness. *Child Care Health Dev*, **30**, 139–50.

Siegel JM. (2001). The REM sleep-memory consolidation hypothesis. *Science*, **294**, 1058–63.

Stores G. (1992). Annotation: Sleep studies in children with a mental handicap. *J Child Psychol Psychiatry*, **33**, 1303–17.

Tamminen J, Payne JD, Stickgold R, Wamsley EJ, Gaskell MG. (2010). Sleep spindle activity is associated with the integration of new memories and existing knowledge. *J Neurosci*, **30**, 14356–60.

Vendrame M, Loddenkemper T, Zarowski M *et al.* (2012). Analysis of EEG patterns and genotypes in patients with Angelman syndrome. *Epilepsy Behav*, **23**, 261–5.

Wiggs L, Stores G. (1996). Sleep problems in children with severe intellectual disabilities: What help is being provided? *J Appl Res Intellect*, **9**, 160–5.

Epilepsy

Epilepsy, which features prominently in the neurodevelopmental disorders, is associated with sleep in many ways (Stores, 2013).

Although all three types of sleep problems are commonly reported, there is still a need to improve the detection rate of sleep disorders in children with epilepsy (Jain *et al.*, 2013). Excessive daytime sleepiness and insomnia feature prominently. It can be difficult to account for the excessive sleepiness, and it is thought that some as yet undefined aspect of the basic pathophysiological process in epilepsy must be responsible. However, certain identifiable possible explanations should considered, namely sleep loss, disrupted sleep caused by night-time seizures, poor quality (non-restorative) sleep from subclinical seizure activity, medication effects, non-convulsive status, or a comorbid primary sleep disorder.

The effects of epilepsy on sleep and wakefulness vary considerably with the type of seizure disorder. They can be direct, indirect or a combination of the two. Direct effects are most likely in severe forms of epilepsy with frequent, difficult to control seizures, especially of a convulsive type. Seizure discharge at night can cause many brief clinical or subclinical arousals in sleep ('fragmentation') which impair the restorative value of sleep, adversely affecting daytime function. Circadian sleep–wake rhythms may be disrupted and total duration of sleep can be reduced, both causing impairment of cognitive function and behaviour during the day. Indirect effects can be the result of anti-epileptic medication, comorbidities which disturb sleep, parenting practices, and the psychosocial consequences of a child's seizure disorder including emotional problems.

Although better seizure control is likely to improve sleep, certain anti-epileptic medications have been linked with sleep disturbance. The evidence-based review by Jain and Glauser (2013) of the effects of anti-epileptic drugs on sleep architecture implicates phenobarbitone, valproate and higher-dose levetiracetam as aggravating daytime sleepiness. Insomnia has been associated with phenytoin. Oversedation can be a problem with benzodiazepines which can also cause respiratory depression and worsen OSA which has also been associated with valproate because of excessive weight gain. In general, the more recently introduced anti-epileptic drugs appear to have less detrimental effects on sleep and wakefulness, although some have been associated with adverse psychological reactions including depression which is likely to disturb sleep.

Hamiwka and Wirrall (2009) have reviewed comorbidities in childhood epilepsy, making the point that comorbid conditions can be more disabling than the seizures themselves and may be important determinants of long-term psychosocial outcome. They review physical and psychiatric comorbidities in specific paediatric epilepsy syndromes, and also biological and social factors associated with greater risk of comorbidity. Although sleep disturbance is not mentioned, a number of the comorbid conditions described do, in fact, predispose to sleep problems and their consequences (Stores & Wiggs, 2001). These include varying degrees of cognitive impairment (depending on the type of epilepsy syndrome) which is closely associated with sleep disturbance, and psychiatric conditions such as anxiety, depression, attention deficit hyperactivity disorder and autism. Comorbidity of epilepsy and OSA is emphasized by van Golde et al. (2011).

How well parents cope with the stress that their child's epilepsy might impose influences their ability to promote good sleep habits, as recommended for other children, by avoiding lack of routine, poor limit setting and inadvertent reinforcement of the sleep problem. Depending in particular on the severity of their child's epilepsy, parents' ability to cope can include their fear of nocturnal seizures which, quite possibly, leads to co-sleeping with the affected child (Larson et al., 2012). Epilepsy may also disturb sleep indirectly via the psychosocial consequences of suffering from a seizure disorder (Rodenburg et al., 2011) including the development of anxiety or depression.

Hamiwka L, Wirral EC. (2009). Comorbidities in pediatric epilepsy: beyond "just" treating the seizures. *J Child Neurol*, **24**, 734–42.

Jain SV, Glauser TA. (2013). Effects of epilepsy treatments on sleep artchitecture and daytime sleepiness: An evidence-based review of objective sleep metrics. *Epilepsia*, doi:10.1111/epi. 12478.

Jain SV, Simakajornboon N, Glauser TA. (2013). Provider practices impact adequate diagnosis of sleep disorders in children with epilepsy. *J Child Neurol*, **28**, 589–95.

Larson AM, Ryther RC, Jennesson M *et al.* (2012). Impact of pediatric epilepsy on sleep patterns and behavior in children and parents. *Epilepsia*, **53**, 1162–9.

Rodenberg R, Wagner JL, Austin JK, Kerr M, Dunn DW. (2011). Psychosocial issues for children with epilepsy. *Epilepsy Behav*, **22**, 47–54.

Stores G. (2013). Sleep disturbance in childhood epilepsy: clinical implications, assessment and treatment. *Arch Dis Child*, **98**, 548–51.

Stores G, Wiggs L, eds. *Sleep Disturbance in Children and Adolescents with Disorders of Development: its Significance and Management.* Clinics in Developmental Medicine No 155. London: Mac Keith Press 2001.

van Golde EJA, Gutter T, de Weerd AW. (2011). Sleep disturbance in people with epilepsy: prevalence, impact and treatment. *Sleep Med Rev*, **15**, 357–68.

Sleep related breathing disorders (SRBD)

These disorders are widespread in the field of neurodevelopmental disorders. In ICSD-3 they are grouped into obstructive sleep apnoea disorders (OSA), central sleep apnoea disorders, sleep related hypoventilation disorders, and sleep related hypoxaemia disorders. OSA disorders, the SRBD most relevent to the neurodevelopmental disorders reviewed in Chapter 4, are separated in ICSD-3 into adult and paediatric categories because of the significant clinical differences between the two regarding aetiology, presentation, diagnostic criteria, course and complications.

Grigg-Damberger and Stanley (2011) describe SRBD in children with Down syndrome, Prader–Willi syndrome and the mucopolysaccharidoses, as well as children with intellectual disabilities and/or cerebral palsy, epilepsy, cervical junction disorders including achondroplasia, and neuromuscular disorders. Craniofacial disorders and sleep are discussed by Ali-Dinar and Ferraro (2011). Chronic nasal obstruction, obesity, hypothyroidism, gastro-oesophageal reflux causing oedema or laryngospasm, and sickle cell disease are other childhood disorders associated with an increased risk of SRBD discussed by Hoban and Chervin (2007) in their overview of the clinical features, diagnosis and treatment of childhood SRBD.

Ali-Dinar T, Ferraro NF. Craniofacial disorders and sleep. In: Kothare SV, Kotagal S, eds. *Sleep in Childhood Neurological Disorders.* New York: demos Medical 2011, 387–97.

American Academy of Sleep Medicine. *International Classification of Sleep Disorders*, 3rd edn. Darien IL: American Academy of Sleep Medicine 2014, 33–77.

Grigg-Damberger M, Stanley JJ. Sleep-related breathing disorders in children with miscellaneous neurological disorders. In: Kothare SV, Kotagal S, eds. *Sleep in Childhood Neurological Disorders.* New York: demos Medical 2011, 245–274

Hoban TF, Chervin RD. Sleep-related breathing disorders of childhood: description and clinical picture, diagnosis and treatment approaches. In: Jenni OG, Carskadon MA, eds. *Sleep in Children and Adolescents* 2007, *Sleep Med Clin*, **2**, 445–462.

Pain and discomfort

The review of sleep problems in paediatric medical populations by Palermo and Owens (2008) refers to many factors that can cause such problems: the underlying disease process, medications, comorbid psychiatric disorders, and also pain in various illnesses. Breau and Camfield (2011) reported both pain and sleep problems to be common in children with intellectual and other developmental disabilities. Studies by these authors and their colleagues indicate that frequent pain, sometimes severe, occurs in 35–52% of such children affecting their daily functioning and contributing to self-injurious behaviour. Breau and Burkitt (2009) have described ways of assessing pain in children with intellectual disability and severe communication difficulties, and de la Vega and Miro (2013) have discussed different ways of assessing sleep in children in general suffering chronic pain. Chambers *et al.* (2008) emphasize the importance of sleep in paediatric chronic pain and the part psychologists can play in this area of clinical enquiry including treatment.

Disrupted sleep caused by various types of pain (including muscle or joint pain, headache or earache) in children in general, or associated with various physical disabilities such as cerebral palsy and muscular dystrophy, has been discussed (Long *et al.*, 2008; Hemmingsson *et al.*, 2009). Children with developmental disabilities and medical problems (especially abdominal pain but also other potentially painful conditions) were described by Ghanizadeh and Faghih (2011) as having higher rates of sleep disturbance than those without such medical problems. The essence of the findings in the detailed questionnaire study of children with developmental disabilities by Breau and Camfield (2011) was that pain does indeed disrupt sleep (especially causing night waking, parasomnias and sleep disordered breathing) even when the pain is being treated with medication, suggesting that the pain management may not have been adequate.

Vendrame and Kothare (2011) have discussed the relationships specifically between headache and sleep. They review the evidence, mainly from adult studies, that, in addition to headache being linked with sleep disturbance (for example OSA), headache disorders (chronic migraine and chronic tension-type headache) can impair sleep quality and cause night waking and excessive daytime sleepiness, as well as altering sleep physiology. Such associations may be mediated by anxiety or depression. A further suggested relationship is that headache disorders such as migraine, cluster headache and paroxysmal hemicrania might be intrinsically related to sleep physiology in that they often occur during specific sleep stages. The authors stress the importance of combined treatment of both the headaches and the sleep disturbance.

Discomfort rather than pain can result from many different medical conditions which may coexist with a child's neurodevelopmental disorder and which require treatment in their own right (Stores & Wiggs, 2001; Bandla & Splaingard, 2004; Palermo & Owens, 2008). Examples include allergies, severe atopic dermatitis, gastro-oesophageal reflux, cardio-respiratory disorders, rheumatological and neu-romuscular diseases including cerebral palsy, and other conditions in which mobility problems may make it difficult to secure a position in bed that is conducive to relaxation and sleep. The management of chronic pain in conditions such as these has been reviewed by Chalkiadis (2001).

The special need, regarding sleep problems, for parental attention at night for children with physical disabilities, especially of a painful nature, has been empha-sized by Hemmingsson *et al.* (2009).

Bandla H, Splaingard M. (2004). Sleep problems in children with common medical disorders. *Pediatr Clin North Am*, **51**, 203–27.

Breu LM, Burkitt C. (2009). Assessing pain in children with intellectual disabilities. *Pain Res Manag*, **14**, 116–20.

Breu LM, Camfield CS. (2011). Pain disrupts sleep in children and youth with intellectual and developmental disabilities. *Res Dev Disabil*, **32**, 2829–40.

Chalkiadis GA. (2001). Management of chronic pain in children. *Med J Aust*, **175**, 476–9.

Chambers CT, Corkum PV, Rusak B. (2008). Commentary: The importance of sleep in pediatric chronic pain – a wake-up call for pediatric psychologists. *J Pediatr Psychol*, **33**, 333–4.

de la Vega R, Miro J. (2013). The assessment of sleep in pediatric chronic pain sufferers. *Sleep Med Rev*, **17**, 185–92.

Ghanizadeh A, Faqhih M. (2011). The impact of general medical condition on sleep in children with mental retardation. *Sleep Breath*, **15**, 57–62.

Hemmingsson H, Stenhammar AM, Paulsson K. (2009). Sleep problems and the need for night-time attention in children with physical disabilities. *Child Care Health Dev*, **35**, 89–95.

Long AC, Krishnamurthy V, Palermo TM. (2008). Sleep disturbances in school-age children with chronic pain. *J Pediatr Psychol*, **33**, 258–68.

Palermo TM, Owens J. (2008). Introduction to special issue: Sleep in pediatric medical populations. *J Pediatr Psychol*, **33**, 227–31.

Stores G, Wiggs L, eds. *Sleep Disturbance in Children and Adolescents with Disorders of Development: its Significance and Management.* Clinics in Developmental Medicine No. 155. London: Mac Keith Press 2001.

Vendrame M, Kothare SV. Sleep and headaches. In: Kothare SV, Kotagal S, eds. *Sleep in Childhood Neurological Disorders.* New York: demos Medical 2011, 367–80.

Obesity

What is considered to be the current epidemic of obesity affects not only adults but increasingly also children, including those of an early age (Halfon *et al.*, 2013). Obesity predisposes to various medical and psychological problems (Pulgarón, 2013) many of which are likely to disturb sleep.

As discussed in Chapter 1, obesity is also linked more directly with OSA (Kohler *et al.*, 2008) and a reduction in the amount of sleep (Bayer *et al.*, 2009) both of which are likely to adversely affect cognitive function and behaviour. Of relevance to the reviews in Chapter 4, childhood obesity has been associated with intellectual disability in general (Rimmer *et al.*, 2010) and, more specifically, with various individual neurodevelopmental disorders, not only Prader–Willi syndrome (Bruni *et al.*, 2010) but also Down syndrome (Murray & Ryan-Krause, 2010), fragile X syndrome (Raspa *et al.*, 2010), autism spectrum disorders (Egan *et al.*, 2013) and attention deficit hyperactivity disorder (Yang *et al.*, 2013). McLennan *et al.* (2011) have discussed the possible role of medication for fragile X syndrome (including atypical antipsychotics, also used, of course, in various other conditions) that might lead to weight gain. McGillivray *et al.* (2013) have reviewed parental including socio-economic factors that might be associated with childhood obesity in general, some of which might be relevant to attempts to prevent or treat obesity in neurodevelopmental disorders, but, as the authors emphasize, more research is needed to clarify the issues involved.

Bayer O, Rosario AS, Wabitch M, von Kries R. (2009). Sleep duration and obesity in children; is the association dependent on age and choice of outcome parameter? *Sleep*, **32**, 1183–9.

Bruni O, Verrillo E, Novelli L, Ferri R. (2010). Prader–Willi syndrome: sorting out the relationships between obesity, hypersomnia, and sleep apnea. *Curr Opin Pulm Med*, **16**, 568–73.

Egan AM, Dreyer ML, Odar CC, Beckwith M, Garrison CB. (2013). Obesity in young children with autism spectrum disorders: prevalence and associated factors. *Child Obes*, **9**, 125–31.

Halfon N, Larson K, Slusser W. (2013). Associations between obesity and comorbid mental health, developmental, and physical health conditions in a nationally representative sample of US children aged 10 to 17. *Acad Pediatr*, **13**, 6–13.

Kohler MJ, van den Heuvel CJ. (2008). Is there a clear link between overweight/obesity and sleep disordered breathing in children? *Sleep Med Rev*, **12**, 347–61.

McGillivray J, McVilly K, Skouteris H, Boganin C. (2013). Parental factors associated with obesity in children: a systematic review. *Obes Rev*, doi:10.1111/obr.12031.

McLennan Y, Polussa J, Tassone F, Hagerman R. (2011). Fragile X syndrome. *Curr Genomics*, **12**, 216–24.

Murray J, Ryan-Krause P. (2010). Obesity in children with Down syndrome: background and recommendations for management. *Pediatr Nurs*, **36**, 314–19.

Pulgarón ER. (2013). Childhood obesity: a review of increased risk for physical and psychological comorbidities. *Clin Ther*, **35**, A18–32.

Raspa M. (2010). Obesity, food selectivity, and physical activity in individuals with fragile X syndrome. *Am J Intellect Dev Disabil*, **115**, 482–95.

Rimmer JH, Yamaki K, Lowry BM, Wang E, Vogel LC. (2010). Obesity and obesity-related secondary conditions in adolescents with intellectual/developmental disabilities. *J Intellect Disabil Res*, **54**, 787–94.

Yang R, Mao S, Zhang S, Zhao Z. (2013). Prevalence of obesity and overweight among Chinese children with attention deficit hyperactivity disorder: a survey in Zhejiang Province, China. *BMC Psychiatry*, **13**, 133.

Visual impairment

Children described as visually impaired are a very mixed group. They vary according to degree of impairment from slight to total absence of light perception ('blindness'), aetiology, which varies with age of onset (according to Rahi and Dezateux (1998), in Britain the main causes of severe impairment are congenital cataract, cerebral cortical abnormality, optic atrophy, retinal disorders and congenital ocular abnormalities), and comorbid disabilities such as intellectual impairment, cerebral palsy and hearing loss. Therefore, general statements about the nature, origins and treatment requirements of sleep disturbance in visually impaired children are of limited clinical value.

The literature concerning sleep has been largely concerned with severe visual impairment. Stores (2001) reviewed early reports dating from the 1970s (often about individual cases or short series) in which sleep disturbance was said to be very common. Emphasis was placed on circadian sleep–wake cycle disorders (either an irregular or a non-24 hour ('free-running') sleep–wake pattern) associated with severe visual impairment. Overall, difficulties with settling to sleep and staying asleep and a tendency to wake early appeared to be prominent, with excessive daytime sleepiness also mentioned in some reports. Leger *et al.* (2001) described blind children as having higher rates of insomnia and also parasomnias than sighted children.

More recent reports and recommendations have broadly been in agreement with earlier accounts. Wee and van Gelder (2004) described abnormally high levels of daytime napping, unstable wake-up times and prolonged times in falling asleep especially in children with optic nerve disease. The findings in a large-scale study by Fazzi *et al.* (2008) indicated that difficulties falling asleep and sleeping through the night were significantly more common in toddlers with visual impairment (irrespective of whether these were of peripheral origin, or of cerebral origin with comorbidities such as cerebral palsy or epilepsy) compared with typically developing children of the same age.

As in adults, the main aetiological factor in such sleep disorders is considered to be the severe visual impairment itself because (as mentioned in Chapter 1) the main cue (or 'zeitgeber') to time of day or night is light input to the suprachiasmatic nucleus. Without this cue, the sleep phase does not readily become entrained to the 24 hour rhythm of the external light–dark cycle resulting in the sleep–wake disorders just mentioned. Interestingly, this is not inevitably the case as even profoundly blind people may be sensitive to light cues because of the photosensitive ganglion cells, a third type of retinal photoreceptor (in addition to the rods and cones in the retina) which connect with the suprachiasmatic nucleus (see Chapter 1 concerning circadian rhythms). In attempting to establish satisfactory sleep–wake patterns in blind children, it may be helpful to promote entrainment by emphasizing social zeitgebers such as mealtimes and daily social contact, although awareness of them might be limited by severe intellectual impairment.

Additional factors possibly contributing to sleep disturbance in children with visual impairment are comorbid physical disorders such as epilepsy, physical deformity or immobility causing discomfort at night, intellectual and communication difficulties, and hearing deficits (deafblindness syndromes are discussed in Chapter 4). Comorbid psychiatric disorder and inappropriate parenting practices in dealing with their child's sleep problems are further considerations regarding assessment and treatment (Stores, 2001).

Stores and Ramchandani (1999) considered treatment options in the management of sleep disturbance in visually impaired children. A more systematic review by Khan *et al.* (2011) indicated that there was still a shortage of well-designed studies making recommendations about choice of treatment difficult, especially because, as mentioned earlier, children with visual impairment and sleep disturbance are such a heterogeneous group. They concluded that there might be a place in individual children for behavioural therapy for behavioural sleep problems, and light therapy or melatonin in an attempt to correct sleep–wake cycle disorders. Caution was expressed about the use of hypnotic-sedative drugs. To these treatment possibilities can be added other chronotherapeutic measures e.g. emphasizing secondary time cues such as mealtimes and social contacts, as well as help and support for parents.

Fazzi E, Zaccagnino M, Gahagan S *et al.* (2008). Sleep disturbance in visually impaired toddlers. *Brain Dev*, **30**, 572–8.

Khan SA, Heussler H, McGuire T *et al.* (2011). Therapeutic options in the management of sleep disorders in visually impaired children: a systematic review. *Clin Ther*, **33**, 168–81.

Leger D, Stal V, Quera-Salva MA, Guilleminault C, Paillard M. (2001). Disorders of wakefulness and sleep in blind patients. *Rev Neurol (Paris)*, **157**(11 Pt2), S135–9.

Rahi JS, Dezateux C. (1998). Epidemiology of visual impairment in Britain. *Arch Dis Child*, **78**, 381–6.

Stores G. Visual impairment and associated sleep abnormalities. In: Stores G, Wiggs L, eds. *Sleep Disturbance in Children and Adolescents with Disorders of Development: its Significance and Management*. London: Mac Keith Press 2001 120–5.

Stores G, Ramchandani P. (1999). Sleep disorders in visually impaired children. *Dev Med Child Neurol*, **41**, 348–52.

Wee R, Van Gelder RN. (2004). Sleep disturbance in young subjects with visual dysfunction. *Ophthalmology*, **111**, 297–303.

Hearing impairment

Sleep problems in children with hearing impairment have received relatively little attention. As in the case of visual impairment, the term 'hearing impairment' covers a wide range of conditions which vary in cause, severity and comorbidity. Also, hearing loss can be fluctuating or persistent. Significant hearing impairment can occur in a number of neurodevelopmental disorders such as Down syndrome (Shott, 2006), the mucopolysaccharidoses (Simmons *et al.*, 2005) and craniofacial syndromes (Swibel Rothenthal *et al.*, 2012). Syndromes in which deafness and visual impairment are combined (deafblindness) are discussed in Chapter 4.

At least the more severe forms of hearing impairment are likely to be associated with sleep problems for various reasons including those of a behavioural nature, reflecting parenting practices. Although some reports have suggested that psychiatric comorbidity (such as anxiety and depression) is linked with childhood hearing defects, the overall evidence seems inconsistent (Hindley, 1997; Bailly *et al.*, 2003). However, the latter authors point out the difficulties that can stand in the way of adequate psychiatric assessment in such children.

Tinnitus (a sound in one ear or both ears, such as buzzing, ringing or whistling, occurring without an external stimulus) has many causes and is said to be common, especially in children with hearing impairment (Shetye & Kennedy, 2010), although, according to Savastano *et al.* (2009), it can exist, sometimes with serious consequences, in children with no ear pathology. However, it can be difficult to detect especially in children with communication problems including those resulting from intellectual impairment.

Reports about adults, especially those with the more severe degree of tinnitus, have consistently described complaints of difficulty getting off to sleep, waking at night and, presumably as a consequence, tiredness during the day (Folmer & Griest, 2000). Oishibashi *et al.* (1993) described high rates of circadian sleep–wake cycle disorders in hearing-impaired children, possibly because of the absence of sound as an important influence in the entrainment of sleep–wake rhythms. Alternatively, the absence of sound when a child's hearing aid is removed at night may mean that his tinnitus is no longer masked and might then be sufficiently alarming to prevent him settling to sleep or being able to return to sleep when he wakes at night.

Just as tinnitus in adults can be associated with distress, sleep problems and psychiatric problems such as anxiety and depression (Wallhausser *et al.*, 2013; Zirke *et al.*, 2013), children with troublesome tinnitus are also reported to be at risk of sleep problems as well as emotional and behavioural difficulties (Kentish *et al.*, 2000; Kim *et al.*, 2012). Various treatments for tinnitus are described, including masking methods, cognitive behavioural treatment and melatonin (Hurtuk *et al.*, 2011; Kreuzer *et al.*, 2013), but there is limited information about their efficacy in children.

Bailly D, Dechoulydelenclave MB, Lauwerier L. (2003). Hearing impairment and psychopathological disorders in children and adolescents. Review of the recent literature. *Encephale*, **29** (Pt 1), 329–37.

Folmer RL, Griest SE. (2000). Tinnitus and insomnia. *Am J Otolaryngol*, **21**, 287–93.

Hindley P. (1997). Psychiatric aspects of hearing impairments. *J Child Psychol Psychiatry*, **38**, 101–17.

Hurtuk A, Dome C, Holloman CH *et al.* (2011). Melatonin: can it stop the ringing? *Ann Otol Rhinol Laryngol*, **120**, 433–40.

Kentish RC, Crocker SR, McKenna L. (2000). Children's experience of tinnitus: a preliminary survey of children presenting to a psychology department. *Br J Audiol*, **34**, 335–40.

Kim YH, Jung HJ, Kang SI *et al.* (2012). Tinnitus in children: association with stress and trait anxiety. *Laryngoscope*, **122**, 2279–84.

Kreuzer PM, Vielsmeier V, Langguth B. (2013). Chronic tinnitus: an interdisciplinary challenge. *Dtsch Arztebl Int*, **110**, 278–84.

Oishibashi Y, Kakizawa T, Otsuka A *et al.* (1993). Disturbances of sleep and waking in handicapped children (II): Trend of circadian rhythm disorders in deaf children. *Jpn J Psychiatry Neurol*, **47**, 464–5.

Savastano M, Marioni G, de Filippis C. (2009). Tinnitus in children without hearing impairment. *Int J Pediatr Otorhinolaryngol*, **73** Suppl 1, S13–5.

Shetye A, Kennedy V. (2010). Tinnitus in children: an uncommon symptom? *Arch Dis Child*, **95**, 645–8.

Shott SR. (2006). Down syndrome: common otolaryngologic manifestations. *Am J Med Genet C Semin Med Genet*, **142C**, 131–40.

Simmons MA, Bruce IA, Penney S, Wraith E, Rothera MP. (2005). Otorhinolaryngological manifestations of the mucopolysaccharidoses. *Int J Pediatr Otorhinolaryngol*, **69**, 589–95.

Swibel Rothenthal LH, Caballero N, Drake AF. (2012). Otolaryngologic manifestations of craniofacial syndromes. *Otolaryngol Clin North Am*, **45**, 557–77.

Wallhausser-Franke E, Schredl M, Delb W. (2013). Tinnitus and insomnia: is hyperarousal the common denominator? *Sleep Med Rev*, **17**, 65–74.

Zirke N, Seydel C, Szczepek AJ *et al.* (2013). Psychological morbidity in patients with chronic tinnitus: analysis and comparison with chronic pain, asthma or atopic dermatitis patients. *Qual Life Res*, **22**, 263–72.

Psychiatric disorders

As stated at the start of the book, 'neuropsychiatric disorders' can be considered as a subset of neurodevelopmental disorders because of the essentially neurological nature of their dysfunction. For that reason, despite the fact that predominantly they attend child psychiatric rather than neurological services, children with autism spectrum disorder, attention deficit hyperactivity disorder or Tourette syndrome are included in Chapter 4 as further examples of specific neurodevelopmental disorders. Although they have some degree of physiological underpinning, the following child psychiatric disorders cannot be regarded as neuropsychiatric in the same sense and are viewed as conditions which are often comorbid with neurodevelopmental disorders. Only the most common examples of this are considered here by means of a limited number of references selected from the many publications on the topic of sleep and child psychiatric conditions.

More detailed accounts of sleep disturbance in general child psychiatric disorders can be found elsewhere (Ivanenko & Johnson, 2008; Alfano & Gamble, 2009). The range of sleep disturbances associated with these disorders is wide, covering all three basic types of sleep problem: insomnia, hypersomnia and parasomnias. Owens *et al.* (2010) discuss the widespread use of psychotropic medications for insomnia in children and adolescents with various psychiatric problems (the appropriateness of which is open to doubt). Kotagal (2009) has described the close relationships of hypersomnia in children and adolescents with psychiatric disorders. The high rates of mental disorder in children and adolescents with intellectual disability have been discussed by Emerson and Hatton (2007), and Einfeld *et al.* (2011). The relationships between psychiatric disorders and sleep disturbances are bi-directional in that psychiatric conditions are commonly complicated by disturbed sleep which can cause psychological problems including those of psychiatric proportions.

Choice of treatment for the sleep disturbance depends on the nature and origin of the specific sleep disorder. Similarly, the psychiatric treatment can be chosen from the array of possibilities used in child and adolescent psychiatry such as behavioural therapy, specific medication and support for the family. A general point made is the advisability of treating both the sleep problem and the coexisting psychiatric disorder simultaneously.

Anxiety disorders

Being anxious at times is part of normal experience at any age. However, the term 'anxiety disorder' refers to something more serious than this. Anxiety disorders are common in children in general and possibly more so in children with a neurodevelopmental disorder. Clinical types include generalized anxiety disorder, separation anxiety disorder, panic disorder, social or specific phobias, obsessive compulsive disorder, and post-traumatic disorder. Combinations of these types may occur and anxiety may coexist with depression.

Alfano *et al.* (2007), and Ivanenko and Johnson (2008) have described the various sleep disturbances reported in children with anxiety disorders. Chorney *et al.* (2008) have discussed the interplay between childhood sleep disturbance and both anxiety and depression, raising issues relevant to future research aimed at clarifying the complexities involved. The most common sleep problems include bedtime refusal, difficulty getting to sleep, frequent awakening at night, insisting on sleeping with parents, and nightmares. Fear of the dark or of being alone is often at the basis of these problems. Nighttime fears are common from early childhood (Kushnir & Sadeh, 2011). They may impair sleep quality but are usually transient. They need special attention if they are intense and persistent (King *et al.*, 1997). Sleep related problems have been described in children with obsessive compulsive disorder with improvement following behavioural treatment (Storch *et al.*, 2008). Sleep disturbances including recurrent nightmares are a frequent feature of childhood PTSD (Kovachy *et al.*, 2013). It is important not to mistake childhood panic attacks (Sinclair *et al.*, 2007) for other types of dramatic parasomnias. Inappropriate parenting style and practices including family disorganization and parental mental health problems can play a part in the development of childhood anxiety states. Other aspects of anxiety caused by stress and trauma have been discussed by Sadeh (2001).

Treatment approaches to sleep problems in anxious children have been described by Garland (2001). These are basically the same as in other children.

They include parent education in ways of promoting satisfactory sleep habits in their child (including sleep hygiene measures), and formal behavioural methods if necessary. Various pharmacological interventions are also discussed as possibly appropriate in severe anxiety disorders where behavioural methods alone have been ineffective. Family therapy might also be required.

Depressive disorders

Just as being anxious in certain circumstances is usually normal, so is feeling sad or having a depressed mood at times, but pervasive depressed mood which seriously impairs everyday living is an illness. Dahl and Lewin (2001) have discussed this degree of depression which they classified into three categories: major depressive disorder with persistence of various depressive experiences or behaviours to a serious degree, dysthymic disorder involving chronic and irritable mood without evidence of major depressive disorder, and bipolar affective disorder in which periods of depressed mood alternate with periods of mania or hypomania.

Main points made by these authors and others such as Liu *et al.* (2007), Ivanenko and Johnson (2008), and Alfano and Gamble (2009) are as follows. The disturbed mood of depressed children is often accompanied by bodily complaints, reduced educational performance, apathy, social withdrawal, difficult behaviour and negative thoughts about themselves or their future or, in severe cases, psychotic features (hallucinations and/or delusions). Anxiety symptoms are also common, and depressed adolescents often have suicidal ideas.

In addition, sleep disturbance is frequently a feature of depressive disorders in children and adolescents. Depressive ruminations, negative thoughts and worry cause heightened arousal and difficulty getting to sleep as well as returning to sleep after waking during the night. Early morning waking is a classical feature which contributes to insufficient sleep and consequent daytime sleepiness with its adverse effects on learning and behaviour including irritability, and worsening of mood. Prolonged and otherwise excessive sleep (hypersomnia) is said to be particularly common in adolescents with severe depression (Ryan *et al.* 1987) who, at that stage of development, are already prone to circadian sleep–wake cycle disorders including delayed sleep–wake phase disorder. Depressed adolescents with sleep problems are considered to be at risk of abusing substances such as caffeine, nicotine and alcohol which can further disturb their sleep.

Bipolar disorder is a somewhat controversial concept in young children. Nevertheless, in descriptions by Ivenenko and Johnson (2008), for example, its symptoms are described as different compared with adults including the occurrence of rapid or continuous cycling between mania and depression, or the two phases may occur simultaneously. In the manic phase, the behavioural disturbance can include periods of agitation, irritability and various forms of disinhibited antisocial behaviour and a reduced need for sleep. In contrast, prolonged sleep, low energy levels, slowing, and possibly psychotic phenomena characterize the depressive phases of the illness.

Seasonal affective disorder can occur in children (Swedo *et al.* 1995) characterized by various depressive features as well as insomnia or excessive sleepiness during the winter months.

Antisocial and challenging behaviours

Various different diagnostic groups are covered by this heading. The predominantly hyperkinetic-impulsive, and combined subtypes of attention deficit hyperactivity disorder fall within this category, but so do other types of behaviour which might be associated with some neurodevelopmental disorders.

The terms *conduct disorder* and, in younger children, *oppositional-defiant disorder* refer to repetitive and recurrent antisocial behaviour of various types. In oppositional-defiant disorder the accent is on aggression and defiance. Sleep problems, including irregular sleep habits, might well be expected in children with these types of disturbed behaviour because of such associated factors as poor parenting, disordered families and unregulated way of life, although such associations are not invariable. However, there have been few studies of sleep in these groups of children, an exception being the description by Aronen *et al.* (2013) of more sleep problems reported by parents of children with conduct disorder or oppositional-defiant disorder compared with controls. Reduced sleep was associated with the problem behaviours. Although Chervin *et al.* (2003) reported an association between children with high ratings for conduct problems and symptoms of sleep related breathing, restless legs syndrome and periodic leg movements during sleep, whether the disturbed behaviour caused these sleep problems or vice versa remained unclear. The same applies to other reports of links between conduct-type behaviours and sleep disturbance by Goodnight *et al.* (2007) and Calhoun *et al.* (2012).

Challenging behaviour includes severe tantrums, aggression e.g. hitting or kicking other people, destructive behaviour, self-injury and other hazardous or difficult to contain acts such as running away. It can occur in a variety of circumstances. For example, it may well be exhibited by children (and adults) with intellectual disability (Totsika & Hastings, 2009). It has also been associated with particular neurodevelopmental disorder syndromes including autism (McClintock *et al.* 2003). Malcolm *et al.* (2012) report how parents of children with life-limiting conditions (mucopolysaccharidoses and Batten disease) describe behavioural symptoms rather than physical ones as the most frequent, severe and challenging to manage.

Self-injurious behaviour is an especially difficult behaviour both to witness and to understand (Symons, 2011). It has been suggested that it is associated with altered pain sensation in some neurodevelopmental disorders (Peebles & Price, 2012). Oliver and Richards (2010) have reviewed its occurrence and treatment in people with intellectual disability, and Arron *et al.* (2011) reported high rates of self-injury in various syndromes, namely fragile X, Prader–Willi, Cornelia de Lange, Cri du Chat, Smith–Magenis and Lowe syndrome, in some cases combined with aggression, impulsivity or overactivity.

Wiggs and Stores (1996) reported more types and a greater degree of challenging behaviour in children with severe intellectual disability and sleep problems than in those without such problems. Parents reported improvements in their child's sleep following behavioural treatment but no objective confirmation of this was apparent. This and subsequent studies (Wiggs & Stores, 2001) suggested that parental attitudes to the problem had changed as a result of participating in the study during which their own sleep improved. Rzepecka *et al.* (2011) studied the relationships between sleep problems, anxiety and challenging behaviour in children with intellectual disability and/or autistic spectrum disorder. High rates were found in their sample for sleep problems, anxiety and challenging behaviour with significant positive correlations between sleep problems and each of the other two disorders. Medication effects did not appear to explain these correlations.

Alfano CA, Gamble AL. (2009). The role of sleep in child psychiatric disorders. *Child Youth Care Forum*. **38**, 327–40.

Alfano CA, Ginsburg GS, Kingery JN. (2007). Sleep-related problems among children and adolescents with anxiety disorders. *J Am Acad Child Adolesc Psychiatry*, **46**, 224–32.

Aronen ET, Lampenius T, Fontell T, Simola P. (2013). Sleep in children with disruptive behavioral disorders. *Behav Sleep Med* Nov 1 [Epub ahead of print].

Arron K, Oliver C, Moss J, Berg K, Burbridge C. (2011). The prevalence and phenomenology of self-injurious and aggressive behaviour in genetic syndromes. *J Intellect Disabil Res*, **55**, 109–20.

Calhoun SL, Fernandez-Mendoza J, Vgontzas AN *et al.* (2012). Learning attention/hyperactivity, and conduct problems as sequelae of excessive daytime sleepiness in a general population study of young children. *Sleep*, **35**, 627–32.

Chervin RD, Dillon JE, Archbold KH, Ruzicka DL. (2003). Conduct problems and symptoms of sleep disorders in children. *J Am Acad Child Adolesc Psychiatry*, **42**, 201–8.

Chorney DB, Detweiler MF, Morris TL, Kuhn BR. (2008). The interplay of sleep disturbance, anxiety, and depression in children. *J Pediatr Psychol*, **33**, 339–48.

Dahl RE, Lewin DS. Sleep and depression. In: Stores G, Wiggs L, eds. *Sleep Disturbance in Children and Adolescents with Disorders of Development: its Significance and Management*. London: Mac Keith Press 2001, 161–8.

Einfeld SL, Ellis LA, Emerson E. (2011). Comorbidity of intellectual disability and mental disorder in children and adolescents: a systematic review. *J Intellect Dev Disabil*, **36**, 137–43.

Emerson E, Hatton C. (2007). Mental health of children and adolescents with intellectual disabilities in Britain. *Br J Psychiatry*, **191**, 493–9.

Garland EJ. Sleep disturbances in anxious children. In: Stores G, Wiggs L, eds. *Sleep Disturbance in Children and Adolescents with Disorders of Development: its Significance and Management*. London: Mac Keith Press 2001, 155–60.

Goodnight JA, Bates JE, Staples AD, Pettit GS, Dodge KA. (2007). Temperamental resistance to control increases the association between sleep problems and externalizing behavior development. *J Fam Psychol*, **21**, 39–48.

Ivanenko A, Johnson K. (2008). Sleep disturbances in children with psychiatric disorders. *Semin Pediatr Neurol*, **15**, 70–8.

King N, Ollendick TH, Tonge BJ. (1997). Children's nighttime fears. *Clin Psychol Rev*, **17**, 431–3.

Kotagal S. (2009). Hypersomnia in children: interface with psychiatric disorders. *Child Adolesc Psychiatr Clin N Am*, **18**, 967–77.

Kovachy B, O'Hara R, Hawkins N *et al.* (2013). Sleep disturbance in pediatric PTSD: current findings and future directions. *J Clin Sleep Med*, **9**, 501–10.

Kushnir J, Sadeh A. (2011). Sleep of preschool children with night-time fears. *Sleep Med*, **12**, 870–4.

Liu X, Buysse DJ, Gentzler AL *et al.* (2007). Insomnia and hypersomnia associated with depressive phenomenology and comorbidity in childhood depression. *Sleep*, **30**, 83–90.

Malcolm C, Hain R, Gibson F *et al.* (2012). Challenging symptoms in children with rare life-limiting conditions: findings from a prospective diary and interview study with families. *Acta Paediatr*, **101**, 985–92.

McClintock K., Hall S, Oliver C. (2003). Risk markers associated with challenging behaviours in people with intellectual disabilities: ameta-analytic study. *J Intellect Disabil Res*, **47** (Pt 6), 405–16.

Oliver C, Richards C. (2010). Self-injurious behaviour in people with intellectual disability. *Curr Opin Psychiatry*, **23**, 412–16.

Owens JA, Rosen CL, Mindell JA, Kirchner HL. (2010). Use of pharmacotherapy for insomnia in child psychiatry practice: A national survey. *Sleep Med*, **11**, 692–700.

Peebles KA, Price TJ. (2012). Self-injurious behaviour in intellectual diasability syndromes: evidence for aberrant pain signaling as a contributory factor. *J Intellect Disabil Res*, **56**, 441–52.

Ryan ND, Puig-Antich, Ambrosini P *et al.* (1987). The clinical picture of major depression in children and adolescents. *Arch Gen Psychiatry*, **44**, 854–61.

Rzepecka H, McKenzieK, McClure I, Murphy S. (2011). Sleep, anxiety and challenging behaviour in children with intellectual disability and/or autism spectrum disorder. *Res Dev Disabil*, **32**, 2758–66.

Sadeh A. Sleep and trauma. In: Stores G, Wiggs L, eds. *Sleep Disturbance in Children and Adolescents with Disorders of Development: its Significance and Management*. London: Mac Keith Press 2001, 169–73.

Sinclair E, Salmon K, Bryant RA. (2007). The role of panic attacks in acute stress disorder in children. *J Trauma Stress*, **20**, 1069–73.

Storch EA, Murphy TK, Lack CW *et al.* (2008). Sleep-related problems in pediatric obsessive-compulsive disorder. *J Anxiety Disord*, **22**, 877–85.

Swedo, SE, Pleeter JD, Richter DM *et al.* (1995). Rates of seasonal affective disorder in children and adolescents. *Am J Psychiatry*, **152**, 1016–19.

Symons FJ. (2011). Self-injurious behavior in neurodevelopmental disorders: Relevance of nociceptive and immune mechanisms. *Neurosci Biobehav Rev*, **35**, 1266–74.

Totsika V, Hastings RP. (2009). Persistent challenging behaviour in people with an intellectual disability. *Curr Opin Psychiatry*, **22**, 437–41.

Wiggs L, Stores G. (1996). Severe sleep disturbance and daytime challenging behaviour in children with severe learning disabilities. *J Intellect Disabil Res*, **40** (Pt 6), 518–28.

Wiggs L, Stores G. (2001). Behavioural treatment for sleep problems in children with severe intellectual disabilities and daytime challenging behaviour: effects on mothers and fathers. *Br J Health Psychol*, **6** (Pt 3), 257–69.

4

Sleep disturbance in specific neurodevelopmental disorders

The point was made in Chapter 2 that, for both clinical and research purposes, there is merit in avoiding generalizations about children with neurodevelopmental disorders in favour of considering specific types of disorder including individual syndromes. That said, not all children with a neurodevelopmental disorder have a specific syndrome. 'Non-syndromic intellectual disability' refers to intellectual disability without characteristic dysmorphic features, malformations or other neurological abnormalities, although such features can be subtle and new syndromes are being described. In fact, many of the points made in earlier chapters about sleep disturbance will apply to both syndromic and non-syndromic conditions.

The conditions included in this chapter are those for which published studies concerning sleep disturbance could be identified. This leaves other neurodevelopmental disorders which have not been studied from this point of view and which await investigation. It seems likely that at least insomnia problems will be identified in children with these disorders, as such problems are such a common feature in the neurodevelopmental disorders that have been investigated. Comorbidities and other influences on sleep are also likely.

The following accounts of sleep disturbance in the various neurodevelopmental disorders differ in length within each subgroup. This reflects the relative attention that seems to have been paid to this aspect of each disorder. The order in which the disorders are discussed is based on the same consideration.

Bibliography

The peer-reviewed articles to which reference is made in the text do not constitute all the publications that might have been cited. Those cited have been selected as being considered the most relevant to the points being made. For the most part, emphasis has been placed on clinical complaints about children's sleep rather than the results of objective findings from PSG in particular, unless such findings are of practical clinical significance.

It will be apparent that there is overlap between different disorders in certain respects. Occasionally, articles concerning adults are cited if they contain findings considered relevant to children. Supplementary sources of information on general aspects of children's sleep disturbance, including its treatment, are to be found elsewhere, for example in Mindell and Owens (2010) and Kotagal (2012).

The opening paragraphs of the accounts of the individual neurodevelopmental disorders, containing information about main general features, genetic factors and prevalence rates etc., do not include references which can be obtained from such general sources as Gilbert (2000), O'Brien (2011), and Hansen and Rogers (2013).

As mentioned in Chapter 2, research on sleep aspects of neurodevelopmental disorders has not only been limited, the value of some reports has been restricted by shortcomings in research methodology. For example, diagnostic criteria and the size and nature of the samples studied may be different from one report to another, and comorbidity considerations have not been given the attention they deserve in assessment and treatment. Rather than confining the following accounts to the limited number of studies that had achieved the more satisfactory levels of research design, from the reports identified by the literature search, a more general coverage of them concerning sleep aspects of each neurodevelopmental disorder has been provided. This need not undermine the value of the overall information currently available. It is simply that often this information cannot be considered definitive. Instead, it can be regarded as raising important clinical possibilities to be revised, as necessary, in the light of further research findings.

Except for the neurodevelopmental disorders about which relatively little has been published concerning associated sleep disturbance, each account generally consists of the following sequence:

- General description of the neurodevelopmental disorder (excluding a detailed account of assessment and treatment of the disorder itself, which would be beyond the scope of the book)
- Occurrence of sleep disturbance in that disorder
- Types of sleep disturbance reported in that disorder
- Factors which potentially contribute to the sleep disturbances (these varying somewhat with each disorder)
  - pathophysiological
  - physical comorbidities
  - psychiatric comorbidities
  - medication effects
  - parental factors (which almost invariably apply to each disorder)
  - other (if any)
- Assessment issues
- Aspects of the management of the sleep disturbances

Regarding the last two items in particular, reference is often made to earlier chapters. As mentioned previously, some degree of repetition from one neurodevelopmental disorder to another is inevitable. Where there is little in the literature about sleep disturbances in the particular neurodevelopmental disorders, it might be reasonable to assume that further study would have demonstrated that such disturbances (mainly forms of insomnia) occur in a high proportion of children because of the likely presence of associated factors which predispose to disordered sleep.

Gilbert P. *A–Z of Syndromes and Inherited Disorders*, 3rd edn. Cheltenham: Nelson Thornes 2000.

Hansen RL, Rogers SJ, eds. *Autism and Other Neurodevelopmental Disorders*. Arlington VA: American Psychiatric Publishing 2013.

Kotagal S. (2012). Treatment of dyssomnias and parasomnias in childhood. *Curr Treat Options Neuro*, **14**, 630–49.

O'Brien G. *Behavioural Phenotypes*. Cambridge: Cambridge University Press 2011.

Mindell JA, Owens JA. *A Clinical Guide to Pediatric Sleep. Diagnosis and Management of Sleep Problems*, 2nd edn. Philadelphia: Lippincott Williams and Wilkins 2010.

Neurodevelopmental syndromes

Down syndrome (DS)

Down syndrome is one of the neurodevelopmental disorders that have received most attention regarding associated sleep disturbance. The condition is the most commonly identified genetic cause of intellectual disability. It occurs once in approximately every 700 births, the incidence being more likely with increasing maternal age, and is caused by the presence of all or part of a third copy of chromosome 21 ('trisomy 21'). The range of intellectual disability is wide with a minority of children falling within the normal intellectual range.

Box 5   Down syndrome

John Langdon Down (1828–1896) was an English physician best known for his characterization in 1866 of the relatively common neurodevelopmental disorder now called, in acknowledgement of his work, Down syndrome. Subsequently, further aspects of the condition were clarified, including the discovery by Lejeune in 1959 that Down syndrome was the result of an extra copy of chromosome 21, hence 'trisomy 21'. However, there is reason to believe that Down syndrome has existed from prehistoric times and that the physical features of the condition were recognized long ago as portrayed in certain historical works of art.

Thousand-year-old skeletal remains are reported to have Down syndrome-like characteristics, and terracotta figurines from certain past South American civilizations appear to depict facial features suggestive of the condition. Nearer in time, some fifteenth to sixteenth century European paintings, such as the Flemish painting *The Adoration of the Christ Child* by Jan Joest of Kalkar (1515), include characters who appear to have the typical facial features of Down syndrome. These findings argue in favour of the condition having affected mankind throughout the ages.

Starbuck JM. (2011). On the antiquity of trisomy 21: moving towards a quantitative diagnosis of Down syndrome in historic material culture. *Journal of Contemporary Anthropology*, **II**, 18–44.

Occurrence of sleep disturbance

The review by Churchill *et al.* (2012) included appraisal of the basic research from the 1960s onwards on sleep architecture in children with DS. This was related to the interest in the relationship between REM sleep abnormalities in particular and intellectual disability. From the clinical point of view, parents have consistently reported sleep problems in children with DS. A comprehensive review by Tietze *et al.* (2012) of sleep disturbance in children with multiple disabilities included estimates of the relative prevalence rates in various groups of children with a neurodevelopmental disorder. Compared with the rate in typically developing children, overall rates reported for children with DS have varied from 31 to 54%. This increased rate was generally similar to that reported in other neurodevelopmental disorders but in contrast to particularly high rates in certain other syndromes, notably Smith–Magenis syndrome and, to a lesser extent, Angelman syndrome (see later). A fuller review of sleep aspects of children with Down syndrome is available elsewhere (Stores & Stores, 2013).

Types of sleep disturbance

Richman *et al.* (1975) concentrated on bedtime settling and night waking problems which they claimed were particularly common in the condition. Silverman (1988) drew attention to OSA in children with DS after which details of the disordered respiratory physiology involved were reported by Stebbens *et al.* (1991).

Since that time, surveys have consistently reported the three basic types of sleep problems (i.e. insomnia, excessive daytime sleepiness and parasomnias (Stores *et al.*, 1996; Carter *et al.*, 2009; Breslin *et al.*, 2011). Features suggesting OSA are often mentioned in these series. The review of parental perceptions of sleep disturbance in their children with DS by Rosen *et al.* (2011) also lists difficulty getting to sleep, staying asleep (to which can be added early morning waking), excessive daytime sleepiness and OSA. As mentioned previously, in children excessive daytime sleepiness can manifest itself as disturbed behaviour including attention deficit hyperactivity disorder-type symptoms. Parasomnias, which take many forms, are commonly confused with each other, especially those of a dramatic nature (Stores, 2010).

Factors potentially contributing to sleep disturbance

According to a US National Survey (McGrath *et al.*, 2011), compared with other children with special healthcare needs, those with DS have a greater number of comorbid conditions, unmet needs (including those of a medical nature) and adverse family effects. Developmental and behavioural problems, as well as impaired quality of life, of children with DS have also been reported (van Gameren-Oosterom *et al.*, 2011) The question arises: what other factors contribute to the children's sleep disorders?

Pathophysiological. Intrinsic factors affecting sleep–wake mechanisms in children with DS are undefined. As in other neurodevelopmental disorders, any associated intellectual disability or communication problem is likely to interfere with the child's ability to learn good sleep habits.

Physical comorbidities. Charleton *et al.* (2010) list a total of 44 specific medical problems that occur more frequently in people with DS. Not all of these problems are particularly associated with sleep disturbance but many are (Stores & Wiggs, 2001). They include OSA, cardiac and respiratory problems, painful or otherwise uncomfortable conditions (such as those of musculoskeletal origin or due to skin disease), gastro-oesophageal reflux, thyroid dysfunction, severe visual or hearing loss, obesity and epilepsy. Sleep disturbance caused by some of these conditions is discussed in Chapter 3.

OSA deserves special mention (Rosen, 2011), being reported to be a complication in 31–100% of children with DS. It is considered to be caused by combinations of such factors as midfacial and mandibular hypoplasia, large posteriorly placed tongue, enlarged or crowded tonsils and adenoids, congenital narrowing of the trachea, laryngomalacia, and hypotonia of the pharyngeal musculature. Other factors predisposing to OSA include obesity, pulmonary hypertension and hypothyroidism.

The point was made in Chapter 1 that there are significant differences between sleep disorders in children and adults. OSA is a good example (Marcus, 2000). These differences include pathophysiology (obesity is the main correlate in adults compared with adenotonsillar hypertrophy in children) and, therefore, treatment requirements, and also polysomnographic findings including a greater tendency to obstructive hypoventilation in children rather than actual apnoeic episodes. As in other groups of children, those with DS who also have OSA are likely to have psychological difficulties, both cognitive and behavioural (Owens, 2009).

Central apnoea, associated with significant oxygen desaturation, has also been reported in children with DS. In some of these cases, brainstem dysfunction could be the result of atlanto-axial subluxation or instability.

Largely, the same symptoms and signs in children in general apply to OSA associated with DS, although over a third of children are reported not to snore (Ng *et al.*, 2006). OSA can have many serious cognitive, behavioural and other medical consequences as described previously. These are mainly due to its disruptive effect on sleep continuity ('fragmentation') which impairs its quality and restorative value. However, there is some evidence that the sleep of children with DS is further fragmented beyond that attributable to OSA (Levanon *et al.*, 1999).

Children with DS are subject to the range of parasomnias that occur in children in general (see Chapter 1) but, in view of the prominence of OSA in DS, further parasomnias associated with this condition can be anticipated. This possibility has received little attention in the DS literature. Schenck and Mahowald (2008) have reviewed the range of parasomnias that have been associated with OSA (mainly in adults). Reference is made to OSA triggering arousal disorders (sleepwalking, sleep terrors and confusional arousals) in children. Nocturnal enuresis (Barone *et al.*, 2009) and bruxism (Oksenberg & Arons, 2002) are other possibilities. The importance of recognizing such parasomnias is that successful treatment of the OSA is reported to reduce their occurrence (Schenck & Mahowald, 2008).

Psychiatric comorbidities. Further comorbidities of DS capable of disturbing sleep are those of a psychiatric nature (Dykens, 2007). Examples described in the literature are anxiety states, depression, conduct disorder and attention deficit hyperactivity disorder (Ekstein *et al.*, 2011), as well as autism spectrum disorder (Ji *et al.* 2011; Magyar *et al.*, 2012). Capone *et al.* (2013) reported a link between depression in adolescents and young adults with DS and comorbid OSA. Sleep disturbance associated with these psychiatric conditions are described in Chapter 3 or later in this chapter. It goes without saying that it is important that these psychiatric disorders are recognized and treated in the general interests of the child and the family as a whole, including the effects of improvement in the child's sleep.

Medication effects. This possibility, which applies in all children, applies no less in those with DS (see Chapter 1).

Parenting factors. As discussed in Chapter 2, parents' abilities to establish good sleep habits in their child (see Chapter 1) are likely to be affected in DS (as in any neurodevelopmental disorder) given the above comorbidities and other complications associated with the condition. For instance, daytime behavioural disturbance and maternal stress have been linked with the sleep problems of children with DS (Stores *et al.*, 1998a).

Sleep assessment

As with other children with a neurodevelopmental disorder, it is appropriate to screen all children with DS for sleep disturbance (Rosen, 2011) and to repeat such screening periodically as sleep disturbance might arise as development proceeds (Royal College of Paediatrics and Child Health, 2009). However, the point has been made that OSA is seen frequently in children with DS in whom it is not clinically suspected (Marcus *et al.*, 1991), and polysomnography has been advocated for all young children because of the poor correlation between parental impressions and PSG results (Shott *et al.*, 2006). That said, such disparities between subjective and objective measures may not be invariable.

Although it might be thought unlikely that the physical and psychiatric comorbid conditions mentioned above will have been overlooked, this might not be so. Therefore, the child's overall physical and psychiatric condition may merit comprehensive review not only initially but, again, at intervals. Similarly, the possibility of medication effects needs to be monitored. Although not covering all these aspects, the evidence-based approach for a brief outpatient consultation for a child with DS recommended by Malik *et al.* (2012) is useful in clinical screening for a number of the factors associated with the condition that can affect the child's sleep. These include OSA and other respiratory symptoms, hearing impairment, other health conditions such as hypothyroidism, atlanto-axial instability and cardiac problems, as well as relevant findings on examination. Further action arising from the findings can then be considered.

Aspects of management of the sleep disturbance

Basically treatment of any sleep disorder in a child with DS can proceed along the same lines as for other children (Chapter 1). Weight reduction might play a part in children who are overweight (Murray & Ryan-Krause, 2010). In general, behavioural treatment for insomnia of psychological origin in children with DS can be effective (Lucas, 2002), and initial findings suggest that brief group instruction for parents of children with the condition can be helpful (Stores & Stores, 2004).

Special considerations in the case of OSA in children with DS include the fact that conventional surgical treatment for OSA can be of limited efficacy and post-operative complications are increased in such children. That being so, other, recently developed approaches may be required (Rosen, 2011). Assessment and interventions have also been considered in the Sleep Physiology and Respiratory Control Disorders in Childhood (SPARCDIC) report (Royal College of Paediatrics and Child Health, 2009) and by Grigg-Damberger and Stanley (2011). However, it should be noted that it has been found that some infants with DS outgrow their OSA in a matter of months (Rosen, 2010).

Barone JG, Hanson C, DaJusta DG *et al.* (2009). Nocturnal enuresis and overweight are associated with obstructive sleep apnea. *Pediatrics*, **124**, e53–9.

Breslin JH, Edgin JO, Bootzin RR, Goodwin JL, Nadel L. (2011). Parental report of sleep problems in Down syndrome. *J Intellect Disabil Res*, **55**, 1086–91.

Capone GT, Aidikoff JM, Taylor K, Rykiel N. (2013). Adolescents and young adults with Down syndrome presenting to a medical clinic with depression: co-morbid obstructive sleep apnea. *Am J Med Genet A*, **161**, 188–96.

Carter M, McCaughey E, Annaz D, Hill CM. (2009). Sleep disorders in a Down syndrome population. *Arch Dis Child*, **94**, 308–10.

Charleton PM, Dennis J, Marder E. (2010). Medical management of children with Down syndrome. *Paediatr and Child Health*, **20**, 331–7.

Churchill SS, Kieckhefer GM, Landis CA, Ward TM. (2012). Sleep measurement and monitoring in children with Down syndrome: A review of the literature, 1960–2010. *Sleep Med Rev*, **16**, 477–88.

Dykens EM. (2007). Psychiatric and behavioral disorders in persons with Down syndrome. *Ment Retard Dev Disabil Res Rev*, **13**, 272–8.

Ekstein S, Glick B, Weill M, Kay B, Berger I. (2011). Down syndrome and attention-deficit/ hyperactivity disorder (ADHD). *J Child Neurol*, **26**, 1290–5.

Grigg-Damberger M, Stanley JJ. (2011). Sleep-related breathing disorders in children with miscellaneous neurological disorders. In: Kothare SV, Kotagal S, ed. *Sleep in Childhood Neurological Disorders*. Demos Medical, 245–7.

Ji NY, Capone GT, Kaufmann WE. (2011). Autism spectrum disorder in Down syndrome: cluster analysis of Aberrant Behaviour Checklist data supports diagnosis, *J Intellect Disabil Res*, **55**, 1064–77.

Levanon A, Tarasiuk A, Tal A. (1999). Sleep characteristics in children with Down syndrome. *J Pediatr*, **134**, 755–60.

Lucas P, Liabo K, Roberts H. (2002). Do behavioural treatments for sleep disorders in children with Down's syndrome work? *Arch Dis Child*, **87**, 413–14.

Magyar CI, Pandolfi V, Dill CA. (2012). An initial evaluation of the Social Communication Questionnaire for the assessment of autistic spectrum disorders in children with Down syndrome. *J Dev Behav Pediatr*, **33**, 134–45.

Malik V, Verma RU, Joshi V, Sheehan PZ. (2012). An evidence-based approach to the 12-min consultation for a child with Down's syndrome. *Clin Otolaryngol*, **37**, 291–6.

Marcus CL. (2000). Obstructive sleep apnea syndrome: differences between children and adults. *Sleep*, **23**, S140–1.

Marcus CL, Keens TG, Bautista DB, von Pechmann WS, Ward SL. (1991). Obstructive sleep apnea in children with Down syndrome. *Pediatrics*, **88**, 132–9.

McGrath RJ, Stransky ML, Cooley C, Moeschler JB. (2011). National profile of children with Down syndrome: disease burden, access to care, and family impact. *J Pediatr*, **159**, 535–40.

Murray J, Ryan-Krause P. (2010). Obesity in children with Down syndrome: background and recommendations for management. *Pediatr Nurs*, **36**, 314–19.

Ng DK, Hui HN, Chan CH *et al.* (2006). Obstructive sleep apnoea in children with Down syndrome. *Singapore Med J*, **47**, 774–9.

Oksenberg A, Arons E. (2002). Sleep bruxism related to obstructive sleep apnea: the effect of continuous positive airway pressure. *Sleep Med*, **3**, 513–15.

Owens JA. (2009). Neurocognitive and behavioral impact of sleep disordered breathing in children. *Pediatr Pulmonol*, **44**, 417–22.

Richman N, Stevenson JE, Graham P. (1975). Prevalence of behaviour problems in 3-year-old children: an epidemiological study in a London borough. *J Child Psychol Psychiatry*, **16**, 277–87.

Rosen D. (2010). Some infants with Down syndrome spontaneously outgrow their obstructive sleep apnea. *Clin Pediatr (Phila)*, **49**, 1068–71.

Rosen D. (2011). Management of obstructive sleep apnea associated with Down syndrome and other craniofacial dysmorphologies. *Curr Opin Pulm Med*, **17**, 431–6.

Rosen D, Lombardo A, Skotko B, Davidson EJ. (2011). Parental perceptions of sleep disturbances and sleep-disordered breathing in children with Down syndrome. *Clin Pediatr (Phila)*, **50**, 121–5.

Royal College of Paediatrics and Child Health. (2009). *Working Party on Sleep Physiology and Respiratory Control Disorders in Childhood. Standards for Children with Disorders of Sleep Physiology*. London: RCPCH, 31–3.

Schenck CH, Mahowald MW. (2008). Parasomnias associated with sleep-disordered breathing and its therapy, including sexsomnia as a recently recognised parasomnia. *Somnologie*, **12**, 38–49.

Shott SR, Amin R, Chini B *et al.* (2006). Obstructive sleep apnea: should all children with Down syndrome be tested? *Arch Otolaryngol Head Neck Surg*, **132**, 432–6.

Silverman M. (1988). Airway obstruction and sleep disruption in Down's syndrome. *Brit Med J*, **296**, 1618–19.

Stebbens VA, Dennis J, Samuels MP, Croft CB, Southall DP. (1991). Sleep-related upper airway obstruction in a cohort with Down's syndrome. *Arch Dis Child*, **66**, 1333–8.

Stores G. (2010). Dramatic parasomnias: recognition and treatment. *Br J Hosp Med*, **71**, 505–10.

Stores G, Stores R. (2013). Sleep disorders and their clinical significance in children with Down syndrome. *Dev Med Child Neurol*, **55**, 126–30.

Stores G, Wiggs L, eds. (2001). *Sleep Disturbance in Children and Adolescents with Disorders of Development: Its Significance and Management*. London: Mac Keith Press.

Stores R, Stores G. (2004). Evaluation of group-administered instruction for parents to prevent or minimize sleep problems in young children with Down syndrome. *J Appl Res Intellect*, **17**, 61–70.

Stores R, Stores G, Buckley S. (1996). The pattern of sleep problems in children with Down's syndrome and other intellectual disabilities. *J Appl Res Intellect*, **9**, 145–58.

Stores R, Stores G, Fellows B, Buckley S. (1998a). Daytime behaviour problems and maternal stress in children with Down's syndrome, their siblings, and non-intellectually disabled and other intellectually disabled peers. *J Intell Disabil Res*, **42**, 228–37.

Stores R, Stores G, Fellows B, Buckley S. (1998b). A factor analysis of sleep problems and their psychological associations in children with Down's syndrome. *J Appl Res Intellect*, **11**, 345–54.

Tietze AL, Blankenburg M, Hechler T *et al.* (2012). Sleep disturbances in children with multiple disabilities. *Sleep Med Rev*, **16**, 117–27.

van Gameren-Oosterom HBM, Fekkes M, Buitendijk SE *et al.* (2011). Development, problem behaviour, and quality of life in a population based sample of eight-year-old children with Down syndrome. *PLoS ONE*, **6**, e21879.

Fragile X syndrome (FXS)

FXS is the most common inherited cause of intellectual disability in males (and also the most common single-gene cause of autism) affecting about 1 in 400 males and 1 in 8000 females. The basic abnormality is a mutation in the fragile X mental retardation 1 (FMR1) gene where a DNA segment, the cytosine–guanine–guanine (CGG) sequence, is expanded. The abnormally expanded CGG segment inactivates the FMR1 gene, preventing it from producing a protein called fragile X mental retardation protein (FMRP) which is important for normal neural development. The 'family' of fragile X disorders includes the full mutation form causing FXS and the premutation (or carrier) form due to an intermediate inactivation of the FMR1 gene.

The clinical features of FXS are mainly intellectual disability (from mild to severe), an elongated face, large or protruding ears, macro-orchidism, and behavioural characteristics including stereotyped movements such as hand-flapping, as well as social anxiety. Males are affected more than females because they have only one X chromosome. FMR1 premutation is generally compatible with normal intellect and appearance, but a subgroup has various developmental problems. The recently described fragile X-associated tremor/ataxia syndrome (FXTAS), which can include dementia, occurs mainly in adult males.

Occurrence of sleep disturbance

There have been relatively few studies of this aspect of FXS despite the fact that it is common. Richdale (2003) described parents reporting sleep problems (mainly insomnia) in the vast majority of their children with the condition. In a larger study, Kronk *et al.* (2009) found that parents reported that 47% of the children with FXS had a clinically significant sleep problem despite medication in 19% of the sample. Then, as part of a US nationwide survey of the needs of families with at least one child with full mutation FSX, Kronk *et al.* (2010) reported on the sleep aspects of almost 1300 such children age 15–16 (78% boys). Parents reported that 32% had current sleep difficulties, 84% of these having two or more sleep problems.

Types of sleep disturbance

In the Kronk *et al.* (2010) series, the main sleep disturbance was difficulty going to sleep and frequent night wakings, although restless sleep, daytime sleepiness and (to a less extent) sleep terrors, night fears, sleep apnoea and refusal to sleep alone were also mentioned. OSA was also reported by Tirosh and Borochowitz (1992) in FXS. Hamlin *et al.* (2011) described the same sleep disorder in association with FXS intellectual disability premutation with and without FXTAS.

Physiological studies have been few. Musumeci *et al.* (1999) described various polysomnographic abnormalities including decreased rapid eye movements, increased REM latency and decreased total sleep compared with healthy boys. Miano *et al.* (2008) have reported that alteration of sleep microstructure measured in terms of the cyclic alternating pattern (CAP) might be distinctive of intellectual disability including that of FXS.

Kronk *et al.* (2010) reported that various types of treatments had been tried (including medications in over 40%) with mixed results. The likelihood of sleep problems was thought to be associated with various health and behavioural factors. The authors usefully discuss their findings at length, including the need for attention to more standardized research designs.

Factors potentially contributing to sleep disturbance

Pathophysiological. The possibility has been raised that melatonin production might be abnormal (due to increased activity of the sympathetic nervous system) at least in some children with FXS (Gould *et al.* 2000). Hessl *et al.* (2009) have discussed the variable degrees of intellectual disability in FXS including its assessment

Physical comorbidities. Epilepsy occurs in approximately 10–40% of individuals with FXS (Berry-Kravis, 2002). The seizures are usually generalized or partial complex seizures and they may occur at night (Musumeci *et al.* 1999). Occasionally status epilepticus has been reported (Gauthey *et al.*, 2010). Seizures are more common in those with FXS plus autism compared with FXS without autism (Garcia-Nonell *et al.*, 2008; Berry-Kravis *et al.*, 2010). McLennan *et al.* (2011) have drawn attention to increased obesity rates in young males with FSX with which treatment with atypical antipsychotic medication might be linked.

Psychiatric comorbidities. FXS and autism spectrum disorder are strongly associated. Autism spectrum disorder is seen in about 30% of children with full mutation FSX (Harris *et al.*, 2008) and has been considered to be a sub-phenotype in FXS (Hernandez *et al.*, 2009). Attention deficit hyperactivity disorder symptoms are also common (Sullivan *et al.*, 2006; Roberts *et al.*, 2011). Other relevant comorbidities include anxiety and depression, 'sensory overload', antisocial behaviour including aggression, inattention and overactivity (Tsiouris & Brown, 2004; Symons *et al.*, 2010). Although children with premutation fragile X are mostly normal, a subset are reported to have the same developmental problems as those just mentioned (Farzin *et al.*, 2006; Bailey *et al.*, 2008; Bourgeois *et al.*, 2011). The pattern of such comorbidities vary somewhat from male to female, they often occur in combinations and at least some (such as anxiety and depression) may persist into adult life (Bourgeios *et al.* 2011).

Medication effects need to be considered as in other neurodevelopmental disorders.

Parenting factors arising from the challenge of caring for children with FXS and its various comorbidities are likely to contribute to the difficulties of instilling satisfactory sleep habits.

Sleep assessment
This should follow the same guidelines for screening and diagnosis as recommended for other neurodevelopmental disorders.

Aspects of management of the sleep disturbance
Treatments for the sleep disturbance itself can proceed along the lines appropriate for other children. A preliminary study by Weiskop *et al.* (2005) suggested that behavioural methods for insomnia in FXS (or autism) can be effective. The findings of Wirojanan *et al.* (2009) supported this view. Tsiouris and Brown (2004) and Bailey *et al.* (2012) have summarized the various medications aimed, in a high proportion of patients with FXS, at their neuropsychiatric comorbidities. They and Hagerman *et al.* (2012) hope that other interventions will be possible to mitigate or reverse the basic neurobiological abnormalities in FXS. If achieved, the contribution to the associated sleep disorders of intrinsic influences might be diminished. Other aspects of the situation, such as epilepsy and family factors, will need to be managed in the usual ways.

Bailey DB Jr, Raspa M, Bishop E *et al.* (2012). Medication utilization for targeted symptoms in children and adults with fragile X syndrome: US survey. *J Dev Behav Pediatr*, **33**, 62–9.

Bailey DB Jr, Raspa M, Olmsted M, Holiday DB. (2008). Co-occurring conditions associated with FMR1 gene variations: findings from a national parent survey. *Am J Med Genet A*, **146A**, 2060–9.

Berry-Kravis E. (2002). Epilepsy in fragile X syndrome. *Dev Med Child Neurol*, **44**, 724–8.

Berry-Kravis E, Raspa M, Loggin-Hester L *et al.* (2010). Seizures in fragile X syndrome: characteristics and comorbid diagnoses. *Am J Intellect Dev Disabil*, **115**, 461–72.

Bourgeois JA, Seritan AL, Casillas EM *et al.* (2011). Lifetime prevalence of mood and anxiety disorders in fragile X premutation carriers. *J Clin Psychiatry*, **72**, 175–82.

Farzin F, Perry H, Hessl D *et al.* (2006). Autism spectrum disorders and attention-deficit/ hyperactivity disorder in boys with the fragile X premutation. *J Dev Behav Pediatr*, **27**, S137–44.

Garcia-Nonell C, Ratera ER, Harris S *et al.* (2008). Secondary medical diagnosis in fragile X syndrome with and without autism spectrum disorder. *Am J Med Genet A*, **146A**, 1911–16.

Gauthey M, Poloni CB, Ramelli GP, Roulet-Perez E, Korff CM. (2010). Status epilepticus in fragile X syndrome. *Epilepsia*, **51**, 2470–3.

Gould EL, Loesch DZ, Martin MJ *et al.* (2000). Melatonin profiles and sleep characteristics in boys with fragile X syndrome: a preliminary study. *Am J Med Genet*, **95**, 307–15.

Hagerman R, Lauterborn J, Au J, Berry-Kravis E. (2012). Fragile X syndrome and targeted treatment trials. *Results Probl Cell Differ*, **54**, 297–335.

Hamlin A, Liu Y, Nguyen DV *et al.* (2011). Sleep apnea in fragile X premutation carriers with and without FXTAS. *Am J Med Genet B Neuropsychiatr Genet*, **156B**, 923–8.

Harris SW, Hessl D, Goodlin-Jones B *et al.* (2008). Autism profiles of males with fragile X syndrome. *Am J Ment Retard*, **113**, 427–38.

Hernandez RN, Feinberg RL, Vaurio R *et al.* (2009). Autism spectrum disorder in fragile X syndrome: a longitudinal evaluation. *Am J Med Genet A*, **149A**, 1125–37.

Hessl D, Nguyen DV, Green C *et al.* (2009). A solution to limitations of cognitive testing in children with intellectual disabilities: the case of fragile X syndrome. *J Neurodev Disord*, **1**, 33–45.

Kronk R, Bishop EE, Raspa M *et al.* (2010). Prevalence, nature, and correlates of sleep problems among children with fragile X syndrome based on a large scale parent survey. *Sleep*, **33**, 679–87.

Kronk R, Dahl R, Noll R. (2009). Caregiver reports of sleep problems on a convenience sample of children with fragile X syndrome. *Am J Intellect Dev Disabil*, **114**, 383–92.

McLennan Y, Polussa J, Tassone F, Hagerman R. (2011). Fragile x syndrome. *Curr Genomics*, **12**, 216–24.

Miano S, Bruni O, Elia M *et al.* (2008). Sleep phenotypes of intellectual diasbility: a polysomnographic evaluation in subjects with Down syndrome and Fragile-X syndrome. *Clin Neurophysiol*, **119**, 1242–7.

Musumeci SA, Hagerman RJ, Ferri R *et al.* (1999). Epilepsy and EEG findings in males with fragile X syndrome. *Epilepsia*, **40**, 1092–9.

Richdale A. (2003). A descriptive analysis of sleep behaviour in children with Fragile X. *J Intellect Dev Disabil*, **28**, 135–44.

Roberts JE, Miranda M, Boccia M *et al.* (2011). Treatment effects of stimulant medication in young boys with fragile X syndrome. *J Neurodev Disord*, **3**, 175–84.

Sullivan K, Hatton D, Hammer J *et al.* (2006). ADHD symptoms in children with FXS. *Am J Med Genet A*, **140**, 2275–88.

Symons FJ, Byiers BJ, Raspa M, Bishop E, Bailey DB. (2010). Self-injurious behavior and fragile X syndrome: findings from the national fragile X survey. *Am J Intellect Dev Disabil*, **115**, 473–81.

Tirosh E, Borochowitz Z. (1992). Sleep apnea in fragile X syndrome. *Am J Med Genet*, **43**, 124–7.

Tsiouris JA, Brown WT. (2004). Neuropsychiatric symptoms of fragile X syndrome: pathophysiology and pharmacotherapy. *CNS Drugs*, **18**, 687–703.

Weiskop S, Richdale A, Matthews J. (2005). Behavioural treatment to reduce sleep problems in children with autism or fragile X syndrome. *Dev Med Child Neurol*, **47**, 94–104.

Wirojanan J, Jacquemont S, Diaz R *et al.* (2009). The efficacy of melatonin for sleep problems in children with autism, fragile X syndrome, or autism and fragile X syndrome. *J Clin Sleep Med*, **5**, 145–50.

Foetal alcohol spectrum disorder (FASD)

This neurodevelopmental disorder is considered to be the most common preventable cause of intellectual disability. The term FASD refers to the range of neurological impairments and other abnormalities that can affect a child who has been exposed to alcohol *in utero*.

The term foetal alcohol syndrome (FAS) was coined by Jones and Smith (1973) since when distinctions have been made between full FAS, partial FAS (PFAS) and alcohol related neurodevelopmental disorder (ARND) (Manning & Eugene Hoyme, 2007). Foetal alcohol spectrum disorders (FASD) covers these variations which collectively have been estimated to affect 2–5% of young schoolchildren in the United States and some Western European countries (May et al., 2009). The economic cost to the nation of what is seen as a large public health problem is very considerable (Lupton et al., 2004). Nevertheless, it is felt that both the general public and healthcare professionals are insufficiently aware of the magnitude of the problem of FASD and its consequences (O'Leary, 2004).

FAS is the most severe end of the spectrum with the complete phenotype comprising characteristic facial abnormalities, growth retardation, and physical and behavioural developmental abnormalities. For the diagnosis of PFAS, facial abnormalities or growth failure can be less, and in ARND the emphasis is on evidence of central nervous system damage following prenatal exposure to alcohol. Outcome in FASD is generally poor with problems of intellectual disability, difficult behaviours and limited psychosocial prospects persisting into adult life (Spohr et al., 2007). Such sleep disturbances as have been reported are likely to have contributed to this prognosis; conversely the problems just mentioned are very likely to have added to any persistent pre-existing sleep problems.

Occurrence of sleep disturbance
There have been relatively few studies of sleep disturbances in children with FASD. Those that have been reported have varied in size, age, possible selection bias, diagnostic criteria and use of terms, assessment methods, control comparisons and other methodological respects, preventing any precise conclusions being reached. However, based on their combined clinical experience, Jan et al. (2010) emphasized their impression that severe and persistent sleep difficulties are frequently associated with FASD. Goril (2011) reported that almost 80% of her series of children with FASD had at least one sleep disorder according to their parents, a rate which was echoed in the findings of Chen et al. (2012).

Types of sleep disturbance
On the basis of electroencephalography, video recording and actometry findings, Troese et al. (2008) described a variety of features in infants 6–8 weeks old born to mothers who had consumed alcohol while pregnant. These included night waking, sleep fragmentation, poor alertness and irritability, and decreased active (REM type) sleep. Stade et al. (2008), having used a sleep questionnaire for use with caregivers reported several types of sleep problems and disorders in a group of 5–8-year-olds with FASD, namely repeated night waking, sleep terrors, sleepwalking and daytime 'fatigue'. Goril (2011) described insomnia, OSA, REM and NREM parasomnias, and delayed sleep–wake phase disorder, as well as fragmented sleep, in their sample at a higher rate than in published normal samples. Chen et al. (2012), having used the Children's Sleep Habits Questionnaire for parents, reported that insomnia of various forms featured prominently but sleep anxiety, daytime

sleepiness, sleep disordered breathing and parasomnias were also mentioned, as well as fragmented sleep in electroencephalographic recordings taken in a subset of the sample.

Factors potentially contributing to sleep disturbance

Pathophysiology. Reference has been made to sleep disturbance (along with other difficulties) from infancy (Burd & Wilson, 2004). Depending on the severity of central nervous system damage, the aetiology of the sleep disturbance in FASD can be expected to include damage to brain structures and systems concerning sleep caused by the prenatal alcohol exposure (Guerri *et al.*, 2009). For example, since experimental animal studies of the effects of exposure to alcohol in early development indicate disruption of the body clock system (Spanagel *et al.*, 2005), potentially serious circadian sleep–wake cycle disorders can be anticipated from an early age, as in the infants studied by Troese *et al.* (2008) just mentioned.

Wengel *et al.* (2011) claim that 'sensory processing deficits' are widespread in children with FASD and associated with multiple sleep problems (mainly insomnia) for which they recommend occupational therapy for sensory-based treatment mainly by occupational therapists. Sensory processing deficits is a controversial concept (not recognized in DSM or ICD systems) in which sensory information is thought to be registered, interpreted and processed abnormally, possibly resulting in extreme sensitivity, avoidance of certain activities, agitation, distress, fear or confusion. It has been described in some other neurodevelopmental disorders such as autism spectrum disorders and attention deficit hyperactivity disorder (see later).

Physical comorbidities. Bell *et al.* (2010) have reported that in addition to their various neurocognitive comorbidities (to be expected as a result of central nervous system damage), children and adults with FASD show a high prevalence of epilepsy. As far as was ascertained, various seizure types were identified, each likely to have different effects on sleep (see Chapter 3).

Psychiatric comorbidities. Early reports described a high rate of hyperkinetic disorders, emotional disorders, sleep disorders, and abnormal habits and stereotypies persisting over time in children with FAS (Steinhausen & Spohr, 1998). This general picture has been confirmed by later studies although various degrees of central nervous system sequelae have been stressed by others (Streissguth & O'Malley, 2000). A strong association with attention deficit hyperactivity disorder is a recurrent theme in the literature (Rasmussen *et al.*, 2010, Peadon & Elliott, 2010). The reviews by Rasmussen *et al.* (2008) and O'Connor and Paley (2009) illustrated that various other forms of psychiatric disturbance associated with prenatal exposure to alcohol have been reported throughout childhood and adolescence including anxiety, depression and antisocial behaviour. Stevens *et al.* (2013) have discussed autistic features in children with FASD.

Medication effects need to be considered as possible contributory factors in both initial and subsequent assessment.

Parenting. Rasmussen *et al.* (2008) have indicated the limited literature on effects on the family which is relevant to parenting practices regarding sleep.

The serious effects on the family of raising a child with FASD and their role in the outcome are discussed by Olson *et al.* (2009), and Watson *et al.* (2013) have reported that parents of children with FASD are more stressed than parents of children with autism spectrum disorder. Shortcomings, especially in maternal characteristics and parenting practices, as well as arising from the likely circumstances in which the basic condition has arisen, might well be expected (Cannon *et al.*, 2012).

Sleep assessment

The previously discussed principles of screening and diagnostic assessment should be followed as for other neurodevelopmental disorders.

Aspects of management of the sleep disturbance

Interventions for children with FASD have been reviewed by Peadon *et al.* (2009) who concluded that there was limited good quality evidence for specific interventions for managing the condition and that there was little or no reference to sleep disturbance. Ipsiroglu *et al.* (2013) have discussed reasons why the sleep disturbances of children with FASD are often missed, and ways of reducing the risk of this problem, mainly by instructing parents and healthcare professionals in the basics of children's sleep disorders including their consequences and treatment.

In the absence of high level research evidence on the subject, Jan *et al.* (2010) draw on their collective clinical experience of sleep disturbances in children with FASD and have suggested practical ways in which such sleep difficulties might be managed. Their strategies are largely modifications of previously published sleep hygiene principles (Jan *et al.*, 2008) modified in the light of supposed characteristic features of children with FASD. These features, however, are not necessarily confined to this group of children and may also be seen in other forms of neurodevelopmental disorder.

The authors suggest that, as children with FASD appear to be prone to sensory overload (auditory, visual and tactile), their general handling and environment (including their bedroom) should be designed to offset this problem and the distress that it may cause. Other measures are recommended to combat, for example, their tendency to be resistant to change and anxious, as well as their supposed impaired sense of time and poor organizational skills. Preparation for bedtime and other aspects of sleep hygiene are said to need special attention compared with other children. Melatonin is then recommended by the authors for children with severe neurodevelopmental disabilities and circadian sleep disorders, possibly as a preliminary to, or in combination with, sleep hygiene measures.

Bell SH, Stade B, Reynolds JN *et al.* (2010). The remarkably high prevalence of epilepsy and seizure history in fetal alcohol spectrum disorders. *Alcohol Clin Exp Res*, **34**, 1084 9.

Burd L, Wilson H. (2004). Fetal, infant and child mortality in a context of alcohol use. *Am J Genet C Semin Med Genet*, **127C**, 51–8.

Cannon MJ, Dominique Y, O'Leary LA, Sniezek JE, Floyd RL. (2012). Characteristics and behaviors of mothers who have a child with fetal alcohol syndrome. *Neurotoxicol Teratol*, **34**, 90–5.

Chen ML, Olson HC, Picciano JF, Starr JR, Owens J. (2012). Sleep problems in children with fetal alcohol spectrum disorders. *J Clin Sleep Med*, **8**, 421–9.

Goril S. *The patterns of sleep disorders and circadian rhythm disruptions in children and adolescents with fetal alcohol spectrum disorders.* Unpublished MSc thesis, University of Toronto 2011.

Guerri C, Bazinet A, Riley EP. (2009). Foetal Alcohol Spectrum Disorders and alterations in brain and behaviour. *Alcohol Alcohol*, **44**, 108–14.

Jan JE, Asante KO, Conry JL *et al.* (2010). Sleep health issues for children with FASD: clinical considerations. *Int J Pediatr*, doi:10.1155/2010/639048.

Jan JE, Owens JA, Weiss MD *et al.* (2008). Sleep hygiene for children with neurodevelopmental disabilities. *Pediatrics*, **122**, 1343–50.

Jones KL, Smith DW. (1973). Recognition of the fetal alcohol syndrome in early infancy. *Lancet*, **2**, 999–1101.

Ipsiroglu OS, McKellin WH, Carey N, Loock C. (2013). "They silently live in terror . . ." why sleep problems and night-time related quality-of-life are missed in children with a fetal alcohol spectrum disorder. *Soc Sci Med*, **79**, 76–83.

Lupton C, Burd L, Harwood R. (2004). Cost of fetal alcohol spectrum disorders. *Am J Med Genet C Semin Med Genet*, **127C**, 42–50.

Manning MA, Eugene Hoyme H. (2007). Fetal alcohol spectrum disorders: a practical clinical approach to diagnosis. *Neurosci Biobehav Rev*, **31**, 230–8.

May PA, Gossage JP, Kalberg WO *et al.* (2009). Prevalence and epidemiologic characteristics of FASD from various research methods with an emphasis on recent in-school studies. *Dev Disabil Res Rev*, **15**, 176–92.

O'Connor MJ, Paley B. (2009). Psychiatric conditions associated with prenatal alcohol exposure. *Dev Disabil Res Rev*, **15**, 225–34.

O'Leary CM. (2004). Fetal alcohol syndrome: diagnosis, epidemiology, and developmental outcomes. *J Paediatr Child Health*, **40**, 2–7.

Olson HC, Oti R, Gelo J, Beck S. (2009). "Family matters:" fetal alcohol spectrum disorders and the family. *Dev Disabil Res Rev*, **15**, 235–49.

Peadon E, Elliott EJ. (2010). Distinguishing between attention-deficit hyperactivity and fetal alcohol spectrum disorders in children: clinical guidelines. *Neuropsychiatr Dis Treat*, **6**, 509–15.

Peadon E, Rhys-Jones B, Bower C, Elliott EJ. (2009). Systematic review of interventions for children with Fetal Alcohol Spectrum Disorders. *BMC Pediatr*, **9**, 35.

Rasmussen C, Andrew G, Zwaigenbaum L, Tough S. (2008). Neurobehavioural outcomes of children with fetal alcohol spectrum disorders: A Canadian perspective. *Paediatr Child Health*, **13**, 185–91.

Rasmussen C, Benz J, Pei J *et al.* (2010). The impact of an ADHD co-morbidity on the diagnosis of FASD. *Can J Clin Pharmacol*, **17**, e165–76.

Spanagel R, Rosenwasser AM, Schumann G, Sarkar DK. (2005). Alcohol consumption and the body's biological clock. *Alcohol Clin Exp Res*, **29**, 1550–7.

Spohr HL, Willms J, Steinhausen HC. (2007). Fetal alcohol spectrum disorders in young adulthood. *J Pediatr*, **150**, 175–9.

Stade BC, Khuu M, Bennett D *et al.* (2008). Sleep disturbances in children with fetal alcohol spectrum disorder (FASD). *Paediatr Child Health*, **13**,

Steinhausen HC, Spohr HL. (1998). Long-term outcome of children with fetal alcohol syndrome: psychopathology, behavior, and intelligence. *Alcohol Clin Exp Res*, **22**, 334–8.

Stevens SA, Nash K, Koren G, Rovet J. (2013). Autism characteristics in children with fetal alcohol spectrum disorders. *Child Neuropsychol*, **19**, 579–87.

Streissguth AP, O'Malley K. (2000). Neuropsychiatric implications and long-term consequences of fetal alcohol spectrum disorders. *Semin Clin Neuropsychiatry*, **5**, 177–90.

Troese M, Fukumizu M, Sallinen BJ *et al.* (2008). Sleep fragmentation and evidence for sleep dept in alcohol-exposed infants. *Early Hum Dev*, **84**, 577–85.

Watson SL, Coons KD, Hayes SA. (2013). Autism spectrum disorder and fetal alcohol spectrum disorder. Part 1: a comparison of parenting stress. *J Intellect Dev Disabil*, **38**, 95–104.

Wengel T, Hanlon-Dearman AC, Fjeldsted B. (2011). Sleep and sensory characteristics in young children with fetal alcohol spectrum disorder. *J Dev Behav Pediatr*, **32**, 384–92.

Box 6 Foetal alcohol syndrome

There has been debate about whether the connection between prenatal alcohol consumption and serious effects on the developing child has been known from ancient times, with claims that this connection can be seen in the Old Testament and the writings of Greek and Roman philosophers. Nearer our time, in particular from the nineteenth century onwards, the effects of maternal alcohol abuse and a specific pattern of birth and later defects has been clarified, with the eventual elaboration of the concept of the foetal alcohol syndrome.

It has been said that it is almost *de rigeur* to begin any lecture on this topic with a slide of *Gin Lane* by William Hogarth (1697–1764) because it has been so closely associated with the condition and its history (Abel, 2001). Hogarth was drawing attention to the evils of the eighteenth-century 'gin epidemic' in London which was considered to be destroying the health of the poor, including mothers and their children, and causing dreadful social consequences in general.

Doubts have been expressed whether Hogarth was aware specifically of the precise and wide-ranging prenatal effects on children of their mothers' alcohol abuse. However, various commentators have claimed that some of the facial stigmata of the foetal alcohol syndrome are recognizable in the child in the centre of the picture falling from the stupefied woman's arms. All things considered, Abel is of the opinion that Hogarth had no personal knowledge of foetal alcohol syndrome effects and that *Gin Lane* simply portrays the neglect and abuse suffered by infants at the hands of their drunken nurses.

Abel EL. (2001). *Gin Lane*: Did Hogarth know about fetal alcohol syndrome? *Alcohol Alcohol*, **36**, 131–4.

Angelman syndrome (AS)

Angelman syndrome is a neurogenetic disorder clinically characterized by jerky movements (especially hand-flapping), frequent laughter or smiling, a happy demeanour and dysmorphic facial features, in association with seizures, developmental delay and intellectual disability, speech and language impairment, ataxia and sleep disturbance. It is usually caused by deletion or inactivation of the maternally inherited chromosome 15q 11–13 (as in Prader–Willi syndrome). AS occurs in 1 in 12,000–20,000 individuals and is estimated to account for up to 6% of all children presenting with severe intellectual impairment and epilepsy

Occurrence of sleep disturbance
A detailed account of AS, including chapters on sleep and behaviour, is provided by Dan (2008). Based on parental reports, the estimated prevalence of sleep disturbance has varied up to 80%, with highest rates seen in younger children and sometimes improvement in adolescence (Williams *et al.*, 2006). In keeping with this, Richdale and Schreck (2009) described sleep disturbance (mainly insomnia) as occurring in approximately 70% of children with autism spectrum disorder.

Types of sleep disturbance
Reports, such as those by Didden *et al.* (2004), Walz *et al.* (2005), Williams *et al.* (2006) and Pelc *et al.* (2008), indicate that the sleep problem most consistently described by parents and caregivers is insomnia mainly taking the usual forms of difficulty settling to sleep at bedtime and frequent troublesome night waking, but also seemingly less need for sleep than other children resulting in early morning waking. However, attention has also been drawn to OSA and periodic limb movements in sleep (Miano *et al.*, 2005), both predisposing to daytime sleepiness and other adverse behavioural or cognitive effects. The sleep questionnaire study by Bruni *et al.* (2004) added yet other sleep complaints by parents, i.e. restless sleep, destructive behaviour at night, enuresis, bruxism, sleepwalking, sleep terrors and sleep paralysis.

Factors potentially contributing to sleep disturbance
Pathophysiological. The widespread neuropathological changes in brain structure and function that are being demonstrated (Dan, 2009) might well be relevant, and the affected child may fail to acquire good sleep habits because of cognitive limitations. Also intrinsic melatonin abnormalities in AS have been suggested by Braam *et al.* (2008).

Physical comorbidities. The many possible comorbidities in AS have been discussed by Thibert *et al.* (2013). Epilepsy is the most notable physical comorbid condition in children with AS (Valente *et al.*, 2006; Pelc *et al.*, 2008; Conant *et al.*, 2009; Fiumara *et al.*, 2010). It is often severe and difficult to control. Onset of seizures occurs in less than 25% of children in the first year but in 85% by the age of 3. The following types of seizures occur, often in combination: atypical absences, generalized tonic-clonic, atonic, myoclonic including myoclonic status epilepticus, and partial and non-convulsive status epilepticus. Certain electroencephalographic features, including various types of rhythmic slow activity sometimes with spikes or sharp waves (Vendrame *et al.*, 2012), are not diagnostic but can be suggestive of AS at an early age.

'Sensory processing abnormalities' (a concept of uncertain validity; see discussion under foetal alcohol spectrum disorder above) in children and young adults with AS have been reported by Walz and Baranek (2006) who also discuss intervention approaches.

Psychiatric comorbidities. Despite the positive demeanour which forms part of the behavioural phenotype of AS (Williams, 2010), preliminary reports (Summers *et al.*, 1995; Clarke & Marston, 2000; Barry *et al.*, 2005) suggest a number of problem behaviours, each capable of disturbing sleep, in some children with the condition: tantrums, aggression, challenging behaviour and hyperactivity. Whether some or all of these have been part of strictly defined attention deficit hyperactivity disorder is unclear because formal diagnostic criteria for this condition have apparently not been used. Autism spectrum disorder associated with AS has been reported (Peters *et al.*, 2004; Trillingsgaard & Østergaard, 2004; Bonati *et al.*, 2007) although the extent of the association is not yet clear.

Medication effects should be considered as in other neurodevelopmental disorders.

Parenting. Griffith *et al.* (2011) and Goldman *et al.* (2012) have described the adverse effects of stress on the well-being and parenting ability of parents of children with AS.

Assessment
In the light of the likely multifactorial origins of sleep disturbance, a thorough analysis of the cause(s) of a child's sleep problem is, as usual, essential including screening for sleep disturbance and, as appropriate, diagnostic procedures as described in earlier chapters. In case the physical and behavioural or psychiatric comorbid factors mentioned above have been overlooked, the child's overall condition may merit comprehensive review, initially and at intervals. Similarly, possible medication effects should be monitored.

Aspects of management of the sleep disturbance
With the usual provisos discussed earlier, use can be made of the various types of treatment recommended for children's sleep disorders in general including sleep hygiene and behavioural methods. Allen *et al.* (2013) found a behavioural treatment package (comprising attention to the sleep environment, the sleep–wake schedule and parent–child interactions) achieved a sustained improvement in disruptive bedtime behaviour and settling problems in a small group of children with AS and chronic sleep problems. As in other neurodevelopmental disorders, the value of medication for children with AS including melatonin is uncertain, although positive results have been claimed with the use of low doses of melatonin in small groups of children specifically affected by AS (Zhdanova *et al.*, 1999; Braam *et al.*, 2008). Individual differences in response are difficult to explain with the information currently available.

Additional considerations in the case of any child with a neurodevelopmental disorder such as AS include attention to coexisting medical, behavioural or psychiatric problems. Attempts to control the child's epilepsy are particularly important because of the disruptive effects of seizures on sleep described earlier. The review by Fiumara *et al.* (2010) of treatments for epilepsy in AS suggests that valproate, ethosuximide and clonazepam are felt to be generally the most effective anti-epileptic drugs (possibly in combinations) whereas seizures may be worsened by carbamazepine, oxcarbazepine and vigabatrin. Seizure control may improve by about 5 years of age.

Allen KD, Kuhn BR, DeHaai KA, Wallace DP. (2013). Evaluation of a behavioral treatment package to reduce sleep problems in children with Angelman syndrome. *Res Dev Disabil*, **34**, 676–86.

Barry RJ, Leitner RP, Clarke AR, Einfeld SL. (2005). Behavioral aspects of Angelman syndrome: a case control study. *Am J Med Genet A*, **132A**, 8–12.

Bonati MT, Russo S, Finelli P *et al.* (2007). Evaluation of autism traits in Angelman syndrome: a resource to unfold autism genes. *Neurogenetics*, **8**, 169–78.

Braam W, Didden R, Smits MG, Curfs LM. (2008). Melatonin for chronic insomnia in Angelman syndrome: a randomized placebo-controlled trial. *J Child Neurology*, **23**, 649–54.

Bruni O, Ferri R, D'Agostino G *et al.* (2004). Sleep disturbances in Angelman syndrome: a questionnaire study. *Brain Dev*, **26**, 233–40.

Clarke DJ, Marston G. (2000). Problem behaviours associated with 15q Angelman syndrome. *Am J Ment Retard*, **105**, 25–31.

Conant KD, Thibert RL, Thiele EA. (2009). Epilepsy and the sleep–wake patterns found in Angelman syndrome. *Epilepsia*, **50**, 2497–500.

Dan B. (2008). *Angelman Syndrome* Clinics in Developmental Medicine No. 177. London: MacKeith Press.

Dan B. (2009). Angelman syndrome: current understanding and research projects. *Epilepsia*, **50**, 2331–9.

Didden R, Korzilius H, Smits MG, Curfs LM. (2004). Sleep problems in individuals with Angelman syndrome. *Am J Ment Retard*, **109**, 275–84.

Fiumara A, Pittala A, Cocuzza M, Sorge G. (2010). Epilepsy in patients with Angelman syndrome. *Ital J Pediatr*, **36**, 31.

Goldman SE, Bichel TJ, Surdyka K, Malow BA. (2012). Sleep in children and adolescents with Angelman syndrome: association with parent sleep and stress. *J Intellect Disabil Res*, **56**, 600–8.

Griffith GM, Hastings RP, Oliver C *et al.* (2011). Psychological well-being in parents of children with Angelman, Cornelia de Lange and Cri du Chat syndromes. *J Intellect Disabil Res*, **55**, 397–410.

Miano S, Bruni O, Elia M *et al.* (2005). Sleep breathing and periodic leg movement pattern in Angelman syndrome: a polysomnographic study. *Clin Neurophysiol*, **116**, 2685–92.

Pelc MK, Cheron G, Boyd SG, Dan B. (2008). Are there distinctive sleep problems in Angelman syndrome? *Sleep Med*, **9**, 434–41.

Peters SU, Beaudet AL, Madduri N, Bacino CA. (2004). Autism in Angelman syndrome: implications for autism research. *Clin Genet*, **66**, 530–6.

Richdale AL, Schreck KA. (2009). Sleep problems in autism spectrum disorders: prevalence, nature, & possible biopsychosocial aetiologies. *Sleep Med Rev*, **13**, 403–11.

Summers JA, Allison DB, Lynch PS, Sandler L. (1995). Behaviour problems in Angelman syndrome. *J Intellect Disabil Res*, **39**, 97–106.

Thibert RL, Larson AM, Hsieh DT, Raby AR, Theile EA. (2013). Neurologic manifestations of Angelman syndrome. *Pediatr Neurol*, **48**, 271–9.

Trillingsgaard A, Østergaard JR. (2004). Autism in Angelman syndrome: an exploration of comorbidity. *Autism*, **8**, 163–74.

Valente KD, Koiffmann CP, Fridman C. (2006). Epilepsy in patients with Angelman syndrome caused by a deletion of the chromosome 15q11–13. *Arch Neurol*, **63**, 122–8.

Vendrame M, Loddenkemper T, Zarowski M *et al.* (2012). Analysis of EEG patterns and genotypes in patients with Angelman syndrome. *Epilepsy Behav*, **23**, 261–5.

Walz NC, Baranek GT. (2006). Sensory processing patterns in persons with Angelman syndrome. *Am J Occup Ther*, **60**, 472–9.

Walz NC, Beebe D, Byars K. (2005). Sleep in individuals with Angelman syndrome: parent perceptions of patterns and problems. *Am J Ment Retard*, **110**, 243–52.

Williams CA. (2010). The behavioral phenotype of the Angelman syndrome. *Am J Med Genet C Semin Med Genet*, **154C**, 432–7.

Williams CA, Beaudet AL, Clayton-Smith J *et al.* (2006). Angelman syndrome 2005: updated consensus for diagnostic criteria. *Am J Med Genet A*, **140**, 413–18.

Zhdanova IV, Wurtman RJ, Wagstaff J. (1999). Effects of a low dose of melatonin on sleep in children with Angelman syndrome. *J Pediatr Endocrinol Metab*, **12**, 57–67.

Prader–Willi syndrome (PWS)

PWS is a genetic disorder caused by absent or deficient expression of the paternally derived imprinted genes on chromosome 15q 11-q13 (as in Angelman syndrome). Typically initial features in infancy involve hypotonia and feeding difficulties which may cause failure to thrive, followed later by developmental delays including cognitive abnormalities, together with hyperphagia with extreme food-seeking behaviours resulting in obesity and its complications.

Occurrence of sleep disturbance
The overall prevalence of sleep disturbances in PWS is uncertain but they are considered to be frequent and often multiple, independent of age and weight (Cataletto *et al.*, 2011).

Types of sleep disturbance
In view of the cognitive and behavioural problems in children with PWS, insomnia of behavioural origin can be expected and, indeed, Vela-Bueno *et al.* (1984), in describing the various sleep patterns in their patients with PWS, included difficulties settling to sleep and staying asleep. Otherwise, this type of sleep problem does not appear to have been studied in any detail. In contrast, excessive daytime sleepiness has for long consistently been reported to occur in almost all people with PWS and has been given much attention, especially regarding its aetiology (Camfferman *et al.*, 2008). Vela-Bueno *et al.* (1984) described 'striking disturbances of sleep–wakefulness patterns' in a group of young PWS patients. Excessive daytime sleepiness was a prominent subjective and objective feature as in other early reports (Vela-Bueno *et al.*, 2001). In their series, Richdale *et al.* (1999) and Cotton and Richdale (2006) emphasized excessive sleepiness (more marked than that found in children with Down syndrome, fragile X syndrome, autism and other children with intellectual impairment) which they found to be closely associated with disturbed behaviour. Excessive daytime sleepiness often continues to be a problem into adult life (Maas *et al.*, 2010).

Grigg-Damberger and Stanley (2011) have discussed sleep disordered breathing in PWS. It is reported to be common and associated with the abnormal behaviours described below. Sleep-related hypoventilation, closely associated with REM sleep is the most common pattern of sleep disordered breathing in PWS and is thought to be caused by a primary disorder of ventilatory control. Central apnoea is described and also OSA but only in a minority of PWS patients The possibility of a narcolepsy-type disorder has been entertained but clinical features of the narcolepsy syndrome are not in evidence in PWS and hypocretin deficiency has not been demonstrated in the condition.

Factors potentially contributing to sleep disturbance

Pathophysiological. Parkes (1999) considered the possible neuroanatomical basis of various sleep disorders in certain inborn errors of metabolism including PWS. The aetiology of excessive daytime sleepiness (EDS) in PWS has been a particular consideration. EDS together with the characteristic obesity and noisy respiration in sleep (Richdale *et al.*, 1999) might suggest that OSA is the usual explanation but this has been shown to not be the case in most patients. Therefore, obesity is thought to be a contributory factor but not a sufficient explanation. The weight of opinion is that, in most cases, excessive daytime sleepiness in PWS is caused by some intrinsic hypothalamic abnormality rather than sleep disordered breathing (Manni *et al.*, 2001) as it often persists after successful treatment of SDB and weight loss. The hypothalamic dysfunction is thought to result in persistent generalized hypoarousal (Camfferman *et al.*, 2006).

Most individuals with PWS have a mild to moderate degree of intellectual impairment (Cataletto *et al.*, 2011) but as in other neurodevelopmental disorders where intellectual disability is a feature, learning satisfactory sleep habits is likely to be impaired.

Physical comorbidities. The possible aetiological importance of obesity in the sleep disturbance of patients with PWS has already been discussed.

Psychiatric comorbidities. Individuals with PWS are described as eventually having a unique behavioural profile which includes, in addition to excessive eating, repetitive and ritualistic acts, self-injurious behaviours such as skin picking, temper outbursts, lying and stealing including in the pursuit of food, reduced activity levels, and mood and sleep disturbances (Whittington & Holland, 2010). In addition to the behavioural problems just mentioned, the following psychiatric disorders associated with PWS have been reported: attention deficit hyperactivity disorder-like symptoms (Wilgren & Hansen, 2005), autism spectrum disorder (Dykens *et al.*, 2011), depressive and psychotic disorders (Dykens & Shah, 2003) and obsessive-compulsive behaviour (State *et al.*, 1999). In their different ways, all are capable of contributing to sleep disturbance.

Medication effects. Consideration of possibly harmful effects on sleep apply to patients with PWS as in other neurodevelopmental disorders.

Parenting. Many aspects of PWS, including the behavioural problems mentioned above, impose considerable stress on parents which is likely to impair parenting ability in many cases.

Sleep assessment

Again, the same basic principles concerning screening and diagnosis apply as in other neurodevelopmental disorders

Aspects of management of the sleep disturbance

The comprehensive guidelines for the diagnosis and management of PWS provided by Goldstone *et al.* (2008) and Cataletto *et al.* (2011) include sections on the management of sleep disturbances. Abnormal sleep is said to be an important but often overlooked factor which contributes to psychological difficulties in people with PWS (Camfferman *et al.*, 2006) but the aetiological uncertainties about the sleep disturbances limit treatment possibilities. However, obesity and OSA should be treated as thoroughly as possible. Stimulants have been used for excessive sleepiness which persists following such treatment but this has not been adequately evaluated (Grigg-Damberg & Stanley, 2011). The efficacy of various psychotropic medications for patients with PWS has been discussed by Soni *et al.* (2007). Growth hormone treatment of children with PWS is said to have produced a variety of beneficial effects, usually but not always on sleep (Miller *et al.*, 2006), including improved psychological functioning (Myers *et al.*, 2007). Miller and Wagner (2013) point to controversy whether growth hormone improves or worsens sleep disordered breathing. The treatments of other problems and disorders which can disturb sleep in children with PWS follow the same principles as those recommended for other neurodevelopmental disorders.

Camfferman D, Lushington K, O'Donoghue F, McEvoy RD. (2006). Obstructive sleep apnea syndrome in Prader–Willi Syndrome: an unrecognized and untreated cause of cognitive and behavioral deficits? *Neuropsychol Rev*, **16**, 123–9.

Camfferman D, McEvoy RD, O'Donoghue F, Lushington K. (2008). Prader Willi Syndrome and excessive daytime sleepiness. *Sleep Med Rev*, **12**, 65–75.

Cataletto M, Angulo M, Hertz G, Whitman B. (2011). Prader–Willi syndrome: A primer for clinicians. *Int J Pediatr Endocrinol*, **2011**, 12.

Cotton S, Richdale A. (2006). Brief report: parental descriptions of sleep problems in children with autism, Down syndrome, and Prader–Willi syndrome. *Res Dev Disabil*, **27**, 151–61.

Dykens E, Shah B. (2003). Psychiatric disorders in Prader–Willi syndrome: epidemiology and management. *CNS Drugs*, **17**, 167–78.

Dykens EM, Lee E, Roof E. (2011). Prader–Willi syndrome and autism spectrum disorders: an evolving story. *J Neurodev Disord*, **3**, 225–37.

Goldstone AP, Holland AJ, Hauffa BP, Hokken-Koelega AC, Tauber M. (2008). Recommendations for the diagnosis and management of Prader-Willi syndrome. *J Clin Endocrinol Metab*, **93**, 4183–97.

Grigg-Damberger M, Stanley JJ. (2011). Sleep-related breathing disorders in children with miscellaneous neurological disorders. In: Kothare SV, Kotagal S, eds. *Sleep in Childhood Neurological Disorders*. New York: Demos Medical, 247–52.

Maas APHM, Sinnema M, Didden R et al. (2010). Sleep disturbances and behavioural problems in adults with Prader–Willi syndrome. *J Intellect Disabil Res*, **54**, 906–17.

Manni R, Politini L, Nobili L *et al.* (2001). Hypersomnia in the Prader Willi syndrome: clinical-electrophysiological features and underlying factors. *Clin Neurophysiol*, **112**, 800–5.

Miller J, Silverstein J, Shuster J, Driscoll DJ, Wagner M. (2006). Short-term effects of growth hormone on sleep abnormalities in Prader–Willi syndrome. *J Clin Endocrinol Metab*, **91**, 413–17.

Miller J, Wagner M. (2013). Prader–Willi syndrome and sleep-disorders breathing. *Pediatr Ann*, **42**, 200–4.

Myers SE, Whitman BY, Carrel AL *et al.* (2007). Two years of growth hormone therapy in young children with Prader–Willi syndrome: physical and neurodevelopmental benefits. *Am J Med Genet A*, **143**, 443–8.

Parkes JD. (1999). Genetic factors in human sleep disorders with special reference to Norrie disease, Prader–Willi syndrome and Moebius syndrome. *J Sleep Res*, **8**, 14–22.

Richdale AL, Cotton S, Hibbit K. (1999). Sleep and behaviour disturbance in Prader-Willi syndrome: a questionnaire study. *J Intellect Disabil Res*, **43**, 380–92.

Soni S, Whittington J, Holland AJ *et al.* (2007). The course and outcome of psychiatric illness in people with Prader–Willi syndrome: implications for management and treatment. *J Intellect Disabil Res*, **51**, 32–42.

State MW, Dykens EM, Rosner B, Martin A, King BH. (1999). Obsessive-compulsive symptoms in Prader–Willi and "Prader–Willi-like" patients. *J Am Acad Child Adolesc Psychiatry*, **38**, 329–34.

Vela-Bueno A, Kales A, Soldatos CR *et al.* (1984). Sleep in the Prader–Willi syndrome. Clinical and polygraphic findings. *Arch Neurol*, **41**, 294–6.

Vela-Bueno A, Oliván-Palacios J, Vgontzas N. (2001). Sleep disorders and Prader–Willi syndrome. In: Stores G, Wiggs L, eds. *Sleep Disturbance in Children and Adolescents with Disorders of Development: its Significance and Management*, Clinics in Developmental Medicine No. 155. London: MacKeith Press, 60–3.

Whittington J, Holland A. (2010). Neurobehavioral phenotype in Prader–Willi syndrome. *Am J Med Genet C Semin Med Genet*, **154C**, 438–47.

Wilgren M, Hansen S. (2005). ADHD symptoms and insistence on sameness in Prader–Willi syndrome. *J Intellect Disabil Res*, **49**, 449–56.

Mucopolysaccharidoses (MPS)

The mucopolysaccharide disorders are a group of inherited lysosomal storage diseases caused by various single-gene defects which result in progressive accumulation of glycosaminoglycans in various organs including the central nervous system. Seven clinical types and a number of subtypes have been identified. Phenotypes vary between the different MPS syndromes depending on which glycosaminoglycan accumulates at which sites. Following a period of normal development, children deteriorate in various ways. Hunter syndrome, an X-linked recessive disorder due to a defect in the X chromosome at CXq27-q28, occurs in approximately 1 in 100,000 births. Hurler syndrome is an autosomal recessive condition due to deficiency of alpha-L-uronidase with the defect on chromosome 4p16.3. It occurs with about the same frequency as Hunter syndrome. Sanfilippo syndrome is also autosomal recessive; there are four types each caused by a different enzyme deficiency leading to the accumulation of heparin sulphate mainly in the brain. Sanfilippo syndrome is the most common of the MPS, occurring in 1 in 70,000 births. Morquio syndrome is estimated to occur in 1 in 700,000 births. Its two subtypes result from the missing or deficient enzymes galactose 6-sulfate sulfatase (Type A) or beta-galactosidase (Type B) needed to break down the keratan sulfate sugar chain.

Sleep disturbance

High rates of sleep disturbance have been described consistently in this group of disorders (Colville & Bax, 2001; Cross & Hare, 2013). Of the seven MPS syndromes, the three in which sleep disturbance appear to be most prominent are Hunter, Hurler and Sanfilippo, each of which (and other types of MPS) has characteristic clinical features and prognosis (O'Brien, 2011).

Types of sleep disturbance

Insomnia in the form of settling and night waking difficulties and short-duration sleep problems of behavioural origin are common whatever the type of MPS, but in other respects the nature and severity of the sleep difficulties varies from one type to another (Colville & Bax, 2001). The Sanfilippo syndrome is associated with most sleep problems overall (Fraser *et al.*, 2005).

OSA commonly occurs in MPS (Nashed *et al.*, 2009). Often severe and progressive, it is caused by a variety of anatomical abnormalities that compromise the upper airway, which also might be affected by widespread glycosaminoglycan deposits (Leighton *et al.*, 2001). In Sanfilippo syndrome, as well as bedtime settling and night waking problems, early morning waking and daytime sleepiness, sleep disturbances include irregular sleep–wake patterns (Mariotti *et al.*, 2003) and also, unlike other forms of MPS, behavioural disturbance at night. Colville and Bax (1996) quote examples of problem or strange night-time behaviours in children with this syndrome, namely staying awake all night, wandering, laughing, singing or reciting nursery rhymes. Many of the children slept with their parents.

Factors potentially contributing to sleep disturbance

Pathophysiological factors causing respiratory problems during sleep include those already mentioned, as well as other ENT problems (Wold *et al.*, 2010). Guerrero *et al.* (2006) have suggested an abnormal melatonin output to explain the irregular sleep patterns in Sanfilippo syndrome. Intellectual level varies across the MPS subtype from normal to severe impairment (O'Brien, 2011).

Physical comorbidities. A variety of respiratory problems affect patients with all types of MPS (Berger *et al.*, 2013). Causes include airway obstruction, excessive secretions, frequent infections, skeletal dysplasia (as in Morquio syndrome, for example), organomegaly and neurological compromise. These problems can lead to progressive respiratory insufficiency, severe sleep apnoea and sudden death from central apnoea. Colville and Bax (1996) reported a history of epilepsy in a third of their series of children with Sanfilippo syndrome. Hearing loss is a possible complication in MPS (Santos *et al.*, 2011).

Psychiatric comorbidities. Severe behaviour disturbance, e.g. overactivity, tantrums and destructive behaviours, was described by Bax and Colville (1995), particularly in Sanfilippo and Hunter syndromes. Parents said they received little or no help in trying to deal with these behaviours. Such problems are reported to often worsen as the children's general condition deteriorates as in Sanfilippo syndrome.

Medication effects. As for other children sleep–wake problems might arise following the use of some medications including anti-epileptic and psychotropic drugs.

Parenting. Malm and Månsson (2010) and Cross and Hare (2013) emphasize the stress placed on parents faced by such serious disorders in their children. This is likely to make teaching their affected children good sleep habits all the more difficult.

Assessment

This should follow the same comprehensive course as that for other neurodevelopmental disorders where there is a complexity of possible reasons for sleep to be disturbed. Muhlebach *et al.* (2011) have discussed the often complex types and causes of respiratory complications seen in most subtypes of MPS as well as treatment options.

Aspects of management of the sleep disturbance

Given the particular complexity of this group of disorders, including the diversity of factors that might disturb sleep, unsurprisingly there are no easy solutions to the treatment of sleep disturbance in children with MPS. The survey by Fraser *et al.* (2002) of clinicians' management of sleep problems in children with Sanfilippo syndrome illustrated the uncertainty of how best to proceed. In addition to emphasizing the need for accurate and comprehensive assessment of the nature and possible origins of such sleep disturbance in the individual child, Colville and Bax (2001) discussed the behavioural, pharmacological and surgical approaches that had been tried at that time and the very provisional conclusions that could be reached about their efficacy.

According to Fraser *et al.* (2005), the same still applied regarding Sanfilippo syndrome, although parents were somewhat more positive about melatonin compared with other medications. With the exception (to some extent) of the management of sleep apnoea in MPS (reviewed by Grigg-Damberger and Stanley, 2011), more recent reports have left the uncertainties largely unchanged for lack of adequate research. The general principles discussed earlier, including the respective merits of melatonin and behavioural treatment, apply, as well as the need for considerable family support in view of the considerable challenge to families of the behavioural symptoms of MPS (Malcolm *et al.*, 2012; Grant *et al.*, 2013).

Bax MC, Colville GA. (1995). Behaviour in mucopolysaccharide disorders. *Arch Dis Child*, **73**, 77–81.

Berger KI, Fagondes SC, Giugliani R *et al.* (2013). Respiratory and sleep disorders in mucopolysaccharidosis. *J Inherit Metab Dis*, **36**, 201–10.

Colville GA, Bax M. (2001). Sleep problems in children with mucopolysaccharidosis. In: Stores G, Wiggs L, eds. *Sleep Disturbance in Children and Adolescents with Disorders of Development: its Significance and Management.* London: MacKeith Press, 73–8.

Colville GA, Watters JP, Yule W, Bax M. (1996). Sleep problems in children with Sanfilippo syndrome. *Dev Med Child Neurol*, **38**, 538–44.

Cross EM, Hare DJ. (2013). Behavioural phenotypes of the mucopolysaccharide disorders: a systematic literature review of cognitive, motor, social, linguistic and behavioural presentation in the MPS disorders. *J Inherit Metab Dis*, **36**, 189–200.

Fraser J, Gason AA, Wraith JE, Delatycki MB. (2005). Sleep disturbance in Sanfilippo syndrome: a parental questionnaire study. *Arch Dis Child*, **90**, 1239–42.

Fraser J, Wraith JE, Delatycki MB. (2002). Sleep disturbance in mucopolysaccharidosis type III (Sanfilippo syndrome): a survey of managing clinicians. *Clin Genet*, **62**, 418–21.

Grant S, Cross E, Wraith JE *et al.* (2013). Parental social support, coping strategies, resilience factors, stress, anxiety and depression levels in parents of children with MPS III (Sanfilippo syndrome) or children with intellectual disabilities (ID). *J Inherit Metab Dis*, **36**, 281–91.

Grigg-Damberger M, Stanley JJ. (2011). Sleep-related breathing disorders in children with miscellaneous neurological disorders. In: Kothare SV, Kotagal S, eds. *Sleep in Childhood Neurological Disorders*. New York: Demos Medical, 252–4.

Guerrero JM, Pozo D, Diaz-Rodriguez JL, Martinez-Cruz F, Vela-Campos F. (2006). Impairment of the melatonin rhythm in children with Sanfilippo syndrome. *J Pineal Res*, **40**, 192–3.

Leighton SE, Papsin B, Vellodi A, Dinwiddie R, Lane R. (2001). Disordered breathing during sleep in patients with mucopolysaccharidoses. *Int J Pediatr Otorhinolaryngol*, **58**, 127–38.

Malcolm C, Hain R, Gibson F *et al.* (2012). Challenging symptoms in children with rare life-limiting conditions: findings from a prospective diary and interview study with families. *Acta Paediatr*, **101**, 985–92.

Malm G, Månsson JE. (2010). Mucopolysaccharidosis type III (Sanfilippo disease) in Sweden: clinical presentation of 22 children diagnosed during a 30-year period. *Acta Paediatr*, **99**, 1253–7.

Mariotti P, Della Marca G, Iuvone L *et al.* (2003). Sleep disorders in Sanfilippo syndrome: a polygraphic study. *Clin Electroencephalogr*, **34**, 18–22.

Muhlebach MS, Wooten W, Muenzer J. (2011). Respiratory manifestations in mucopolysaccharidoses. *Paediatr Respir Rev*, **12**, 133–8.

Nashed A, Al-Saleh S, Gibbons J *et al.* (2009). Sleep-related breathing in children with mucopolysaccharidosis. *J Inherit Metab Dis*, **32**, 544–50.

O'Brien G. (2011). *Behavioural Phenotypes*. Cambridge: Cambridge University Press.

Santos S, López L, González L, Domínguez MJ. (2011). Hearing loss and airway problems in children with mucopolysaccharidoses. *Acta Otorrinolaringol Esp*, **62**, 411–17.

Wold SM, Derkay CS, Darrow DH, Proud V. (2010). Role of the pediatric otolaryngologist in diagnosis and management of children with mucopolysaccharidoses. *Int J Pediatr Otorhinolaryngol*, **74**, 27–31.

Rett syndrome (RS)

This neurodevelopmental disorder affects approximately 1 in 15,000 females with a few cases in males. It is caused by various mutations in the methyl-CpG binding protein 2 (MECP2) gene on the X chromosome. Classical features are apparently normal early development, followed by severe progressive intellectual and other neurological impairments including epilepsy. Other developmental abnormalities are deceleration of head growth, repetitive stereotyped hand movements (such as wringing, tapping or clapping), loss of verbal ability, gait difficulties and breathing abnormalities, such as irregular respiration while awake. The natural history of RS is that of particular symptoms emerging at different ages with periods of regression and standstill.

Sleep disturbance

Roane and Piazza (2001) reviewed a number of studies in the 1980s and 1990s which consistently described sleep problems reported by their parents in the vast majority of children with RS. A high rate of sleep problems (over 80%) was found in the longitudinal study by Young *et al.* (2007) but variations were found in some of the problems according to age and type of mutation. Prevalence of sleep problems was highest in cases with a large deletion of the MECP2 gene and those with the p.R294X or p.R306C mutations.

Types of sleep disturbance

The types of sleep disturbance described in these studies were irregular sleep–wake patterns and early morning waking but a distinctive feature on which emphasis was placed was dramatic night-time behaviour including screaming, crying and laughing. Using direct observations of sleep–wake patterns, in addition to delay in going to sleep, night waking and early morning waking, Piazza *et al.* (1990) documented less overnight sleep and excessive sleepiness in the children with RS compared with developmental norms. The authors felt that the sleep problems (especially excessive daytime sleepiness) worsened with age. Ellaway *et al.* (2001) reported that their subjects did not show the age-related decrease in total and daytime sleep time seen in normal children.

According to Young *et al.* (2007), the night-time laughter decreased with age but reported night-time seizures and daytime napping increased with age. Night screaming and nocturnal seizures were not related to mutation type. The authors emphasize the pathological nature of the night-time laughter in RS which was reported in almost 60% of their series. It was felt that it was not epileptic in nature; otherwise its origin is obscure.

Factors potentially contributing to sleep disturbance

Pathophysiological. Roane and Piazza (2001) considered various aetiological possibilities including intrinsic deterioration of basic brain activity as the disorder progresses. Nomura and Segawa (2005) have suggested that the distinctive patterns of sleep disturbance in children with RS might be attributable to abnormalities in the aminergic systems of the brainstem and their influence on other neuronal circuits. Ellaway *et al.* (2001) suggested that the immature sleep pattern they described in children with RS may be the result of arrested brain development. Katz *et al.* (2009) described disorders of respiratory control as prominent in RS, including periods of hyperventilation and apnoeas while awake. Weese-Mayer *et al.* (2008) point to evidence of autonomic cardio-respiratory dysregulation during the night which they suggest might make the patients with RS more vulnerable to sudden death.

Physical comorbidities. Epilepsy, said to develop in 50–90% of cases and often difficult to treat (Dolce *et al.* 2013), is likely to disrupt sleep in the various ways discussed in Chapter 3. Onset of seizures at an early age is associated with greater overall clinical severity (Glaze *et al.*, 2010). Discomfort from physical deformities such as scoliosis which is common in RS (Percy *et al.*, 2010) is likely to disturb sleep.

Psychiatric comorbidities. The fear or anxiety that has been described as part of the behavioural phenotype of RS (Mount *et al.*, 2002) is capable of giving rise to sleep disturbance. RS has been described as one of the several neurodevelopmental disorders with which ASD is associated but, in this disorder, autistic features are transient, lasting only weeks to many months, and although the two conditions have some features in common other features are different (Percy, 2011).

Medication effects. Given the wide-ranging pharmacological interventions that might be needed in RS, adverse effects on sleep need to be considered as an additional cause of sleep disturbance.

Parenting. Parents' difficulties in having to cope with the seriously disruptive effects of RS on the child's behaviour, physical condition and quality of life (Lane *et al.*, 2011; Kaufmann *et al.*, 2012) are highly likely to contribute to sleep problems.

Sleep assessment
This should follow the same rules as those for other neurodevelopmental disorders.

Aspects of management of the sleep disturbance
As usual, a comprehensive approach to the recognition and characterization of the sleep disturbances, including aetiological factors, is required. Because of the complexity of RS, treatment programmes are of necessity likely to be multifaceted. Since the promising report by McArthur and Budden (1998) of the usefulness of melatonin in children with RS, a number of other small-scale reports to the same effect have been published. However, the same remarks expressed earlier about the limited extent of the evidence for the efficacy of melatonin treatment are relevant to RS. The same is true of behavioural treatments, promising results of which were described by Piazza *et al.* (1991). The general principles for the management of sleep disturbance of children in general and those with a neurodevelopmental disorder apply.

Dolce A, Ben-Zeev B, Naidu S, Kossoff EH. (2013). Rett syndrome and epilepsy: an update for child neurologists. *Pediatr Neurol*, **48**, 337–45.

Ellaway C, Peat J, Leonard H, Christodoulou J. (2001). Sleep dysfunction in Rett syndrome: lack of age related decrease in sleep duration. *Brain Dev*, **23**, S101–3.

Glaze DG, Percy AK, Skinner S. (2010). Epilepsy and the natural history of Rett syndrome. *Neurology*, **74**, 909–12.

Katz DM, Dutschmann M, Ramirez JM, Hilaire G. (2009). Breathing disorders in Rett syndrome: progressive neurochemical dysfunction in the respiratory network after birth. *Respir Physiol Neurobiol*, **168**, 101–8.

Kaufmann WE, Tierney E, Rohde CA *et al.* (2012). Social impairments in Rett syndrome: characteristics and relationship with clinical severity. *J Intellect Disabil Res*, **56**, 233–47.

Lane JB, Lee HS, Smith LW *et al.* (2011). Clinical severity and quality of life in children and adolescents with Rett syndrome. *Neurology*, **77**, 1812–18.

McArthur AJ, Budden SS. (1998). Sleep dysfunction in Rett syndrome: a trial of exogenous melatonin treatment. *Dev Med Child Neurol*, **40**, 186–92.

Mount RH, Charman T, Hastings RP, Reilly S, Cass H. (2002). The Rett Syndrome Behaviour Questionnaire (RSBQ): refining the behavioural phenotype of Rett syndrome. *J Child Psychol Psychiatry*, **43**, 1099–110.

Nomura Y, Segawa M. (2005). Natural history of Rett syndrome. *J Child Neurol*, **20**, 764–8.

Percy AK. (2011). Rett syndrome: exploring the autism link. *Arch Neurol*, **68**, 985–9.

Percy AK, Lee HS, Neul JL *et al.* (2010). Profiling scoliosis in Rett syndrome. *Pediatr Res*, **67**, 435–9.

Piazza CC, Fisher W, Kiesewetter K, Bowman L, Moser H. (1990). Aberrant sleep patterns in children with the Rett syndrome. *Brain Dev*, **12**, 488–93.

Piazza CC, Fisher W, Moser H. (1991). Behavioral treatment of sleep dysfunction in patients with the Rett syndrome. *Brain Dev*, **13**, 232–7.

Roane HS, Piazza CC. (2001). Sleep diagnosis and Rett syndrome. In: Stores G, Wiggs L, eds: *Sleep Disturbance in Children and Adolescents with Disorders of Development: Its Significance and Management*. London: MacKeith Press, 83–6.

Weese-Mayer DE, Lieske SP, Boothby CM *et al.* (2008). Autonomic dysregulation in young girls with Rett syndrome during nighttime in-home recordings. *Pediatr Pulmonol*, **43**, 1045–60.

Young D, Nagarajan L, de Klerk N *et al.* (2007). Sleep problems in Rett syndrome. *Brain Dev*, **29**, 609–16.

Smith–Magenis syndrome (SMS)

SMS, caused by an interstitial deletion of chromosome 17 p11.2, has a distinct multisystem phenotype. In addition to sleep disturbance, this includes intellectual impairment, characteristic facial appearance, various specific cognitive and physical developmental delays, and behavioural problems, notably self-injurious behaviours such as head banging, wrist biting, skin picking, and pulling out of fingernails and toenails, and insertion of foreign objects into body orifices. Seemingly there is relative insensitivity to pain. Prevalence has been estimated as 1 in 15,000 to 25,000 individuals.

Sleep disturbances

Since the earliest reports of SMS, sleep abnormalities have been described in most cases.

Types of sleep disturbances

The above reports referred to the usual insomnia problems i.e. difficulties falling asleep, frequent and prolonged night waking, as well as excessive daytime sleepiness. Smith *et al.* (1998) added common bedtime rituals, bedwetting and snoring. Gropman *et al.* (2006) described SMS children generally sleeping 1–2 hours less per 24 hours than healthy children, with increased arousals during the second half of the night. Potocki *et al.* (2000) and De Leersnyder *et al.* (2001) demonstrated disturbed circadian sleep–wake rhythms together with REM and NREM abnormalities. Lloyd *et al.* (2012) described a single case of REM sleep behaviour disorder in a child with SMS.

Factors potentially contributing to sleep disturbance

Pathophysiological. The comprehensive review of SMS by Shelley and Robertson (2005) included an account of the multisystem aspects of the condition indicating the complex pathological processes involved. As just mentioned, Potocki *et al.* (2000) and De Leersnyder *et al.* (2001) described an inverted circadian melatonin rhythm (high daytime levels and low levels at night) which they considered would probably account for the sleep disturbances and might be pathognomonic of SMS. On the other hand, Boudreau *et al.* (2009) quoted cases of SMS where the characteristic sleep disturbances occurred with normal melatonin rhythms. There is some reason to believe that the SMS melatonin anomalies are due to disturbance of the clock gene involved in the generation of circadian rhythms (Nováková *et al.* 2012), the effect being an abnormal sleep–wake cycle. The usually mild to moderate intellectual impairment and communication problems can interfere with learning satisfactory sleep habits.

Physical comorbidities. Comorbid conditions in SMS especially likely to disrupt sleep have been little studied. For example, epilepsy in SMS seems to have received little attention in the literature despite the report by Goldman *et al.* (2006) that epileptiform electroencephalographic abnormalities were common and 18% of their series of patients (which included children) had a history of clinical seizures of various types. Some of the other medical accompaniments of SMS at different ages described by Gropman *et al.* (2006) are also liable to disturb sleep. Examples include gastro-intestinal disorders and otitis media.

Psychiatric comorbidities. Behavioural problems were considered by Smith *et al.* (1998) as the major management problem for both parents and professionals working with SMS. They were described as aggression, attention deficits, hyperactivity, impulsivity, anxiety and the self-injurious behaviours mentioned earlier. Shelley and Robertson (2005) have also reported a wide range of very common and severe behavioural problems associated with SMS many of which are likely to cause sleep problems in their own right and which impose a highly stressful burden on their parents. Autistic-like features have been described in children with SMS (Laje *et al.*, 2010) who may be diagnosed as having autism spectrum disorder or, alternatively, attention deficit hyperactivity disorder, obsessive compulsive disorder or mood disorder.

Medication effects. The usual precautions about medications as possibly disturbing sleep apply.

Parenting. It is felt that sleep disturbance in SMS is particularly stressful for parents and other family members (Smith *et al.*, 1998). The same authors described how parents adopted various means of arranging their child's bedroom in an attempt to make it conducive to sleep and also lessen the risk of injury when awake and wandering about. Nevertheless, for many parents establishing satisfactory sleep habits in their child is likely to be difficult.

Assessment

The preceding account illustrates the need for comprehensive and detailed assessment of sleep disturbance and associated factors in children with SMS.

Aspects of management of the sleep disturbance

Gropman *et al.* (2006) discuss at some length the management of various aspects of SMS including the psychiatric conditions, medical issues and also, to a limited extent, sleep problems. De Leersnyder (2006) described the attempt to correct the inverted circadian melatonin rhythm by using during the day a beta 1-adrenergic antagonist to reduce daytime melatonin secretion, combined with an evening dose of controlled-release melatonin to restore normal night-time plasma melatonin levels.

Medication options for disruptive behaviour in SMS have been considered by Laje *et al.* (2010). In the absence of systematic evaluation of other pharmacological or behavioural treatments for the sleep disturbances specifically in SMS, reliance has to be placed on the general treatment principles discussed in earlier sections. Foster *et al.* (2010) have emphasized the special needs of parents of children with SMS in view of the demands of caring for their affected children.

Boudreau EA, Johnson KP, Jackman AR *et al.* (2009). Review of disrupted sleep patterns in Smith–Magenis syndrome and normal melatonin secretion in a patient with an atypical interstitial 17p11.2 deletion. *Am J Med Genet Part A*, **149A**, 1382–91.

De Leersnyder H. (2006). Inverted rhythm of melatonin secretion in Smith–Magenis syndrome: from symptoms to treatment. *Trends Endocrinol Metab*, **17**, 291–8.

De Leersnyder H, De Blois MC, Claustrat B *et al.* (2001). Inversion of the circadian rhythm of melatonin in the Smith–Magenis syndrome. *J Pediatr*, **139**, 111–16.

Foster RH, Kozachek S, Stern M, Elsea SH. (2010). Caring for the caregivers: an investigation of factors related to well-being among parents caring for a child with Smith–Magenis syndrome. *J Genet Couns*, **19**, 187–98.

Goldman AM, Potocki L, Walz K *et al.* (2006). Epilepsy and chromosomal rearrangements in Smith–Magenis Syndrome [del(17)(p11.2p11.2)]. *J Child Neurol*, **21**, 93–8.

Gropman AL, Duncan WC, Smith AC. (2006). Neurologic and developmental features of the Smith–Magenis syndrome (del 17p11.2). *Pediatr Neurol*, **34**, 337–50.

Laje G, Bernert R, Morse R, Pao M, Smith AC. (2010). Pharmacological treatment of disruptive behavior in Smith–Magenis syndrome. *Am J Med Genet C Semin Med Genet*, **154C**, 463–8.

Laje G, Morse R, Richter W *et al.* (2010). Autism spectrum features in Smith–Magenis syndrome. *Am J Med Genet C Semin Med Genet*, **154C**, 456–62.

Lloyd R, Tippmann-Peikert M, Slocumb N, Kotagal S. (2012). Characteristics of REM sleep behavior disorder in childhood. *J Clin Sleep Med*, **8**, 127–31.

Nováková M, Nevšímalová S, Príhodová I, Sládek M, Sumová A. (2012). Alteration of the circadian clock in children with Smith–Magenis syndrome. *J Clin Endocrinol Metab*, **97**, E312–18.

Potocki L, Glaze D, Tan DX *et al.* (2000). Circadian rhythm abnormalities of melatonin in Smith–Magenis syndrome. *J Med Genet*, **37**, 428–33.

Shelley BP, Robertson MM. (2005). The neuropsychiatry and multisystem features of the Smith–Magenis syndrome: a review. *J Neuropsychiatry Clin Neurosci*, **17**, 91–7.

Smith ACM, Dykens E, Greenberg F. (1998). Behavioral phenotype of Smith–Magenis syndrome (del 17p11.2). *Am J Med Genet*, **81**, 179–85.

Tuberous sclerosis complex (TSC)

TSC is a multisystem autosomal dominant disorder caused by alterations in one of two genes located on chromosomes 9q34 and 16p13.3. Its prevalence is estimated as 1 in 6000. TSC is characterized by tuber-like growths in the brain and other organs including the skin, giving rise to the term 'neurocutaneous disorder'. Its many possible manifestations vary from mild to severe.

Sleep disturbance

Sleep aspects of TSC have received relatively little attention. However, sleep disturbance has been found to be common, at least in severely affected children with TSC (Hunt, 1993; Hunt & Stores, 1994) with comparable results reported by van Eeghen *et al.* (2011) in their study of adults with TSC. The findings in their study have implications for the assessment of sleep problems in children with TSC.

Types of sleep disturbance

Settling problems, night waking and early waking as well as excessive daytime sleepiness are described in the above studies of children. Polysomnographic findings have been generally in keeping with parental reports (Bruni *et al.*, 1995). In the study by van Eeghen *et al.* (2011), reference was also made to OSA and restless legs syndrome.

Factors potentially contributing to sleep disturbance

Pathophysiological. Asarto and Hardan (2004) discuss the neuropathology and neurobiology of TSC. In cases with extensive central nervous system involvement, the possibility exists that brain structures and systems concerned with sleep and wakefulness are affected. Intellectual impairment to some degree is estimated to occur in 50–60% of cases, and specific cognitive deficits, also capable of interfering with the acquisition of satisfactory sleep habits, may be present even if overall intelligence is normal (Prather & de Vries, 2004).

Physical comorbidities. Epilepsy occurs in up to 90% of individuals with TSC during their lifetime (Thiele, 2004). Seizures usually start in childhood initially taking the form of infantile spasms in infancy followed later by various seizure types which are often difficult to treat. Insomnia was associated with epilepsy in the study by van Eeghen *et al.* (2011). The various ways in which epilepsy can disrupt sleep are discussed in Chapter 3.

Psychiatric comorbidities. Asarto and Hardan (2004) and de Vries *et al.* (2007) discussed the various neuropsychiatric problems in TSC many of which are linked with disturbed sleep. For long, autism has been consistently associated with TSC.

The reason for this association is unclear but intellectual impairment, epilepsy and temporal lobe pathology have been considered to be significant risk factors for its development (Bolton *et al.* (2002); Wiznitzer (2004). Anxiety disorder, depression, hyperactivity, attention deficits and aggressive behaviour are other neuropsychiatric problems mentioned by Asarto and Hardan (2004).

Medication. The usual caveat concerning possible effects of treatment (including that for epilepsy) on sleep applies.

Parenting. Again, depending on severity of their child's TSC, parents' ability to cope with the nature and consequences of his condition and to encourage satisfactory sleep habits might be affected (Prather & de Vries, 2004).

Assessment
Because of the possible complexity of TSC, assessment needs to be comprehensive as outlined earlier. The possible contributions to the child's sleep problems of disturbed emotional state and behaviour, medication and family upset in coping with the condition of TSC and its consequences need to be considered in both assessment and treatment.

Aspects of management of sleep disturbance
Clearly, this also may well need to be comprehensive. The general principles of behavioural methods and pharmacotherapy expressed earlier apply for sleep problems and for behaviour and psychiatric comorbidities. Hancock *et al.* (2005) suggested that melatonin might be helpful in children with TSC and insomnia. Treatment of seizures in the context of TSC are discussed by Thiele (2004) and also van Eeghen *et al.* (2011) who express favourable impressions about the value of carbamazepine and some of the newer anti-epileptic drugs.

Asato MR, Hardan AY. (2004). Neuropsychiatric problems in tuberous sclerosis complex. *J Child Neurol*, **19**, 241–9.

Bolton PF, Park RJ, Higgins JN, Griffiths PD, Pickles A. (2002). Neuro-epileptic determinants of autism spectrum disorders in tuberous sclerosis complex. *Brain*, **125**, 1247–55.

Bruni O, Cortesi F, Giannotti F, Curatolo P. (1995). Sleep disorders in tuberous sclerosis: a polysomnographic study. *Brain Dev*, **17**, 52–6.

de Vries PJ, Hunt A, Bolton PF. (2007). The psychopathologies of children and adolescents with tuberous sclerosis complex (TSC): a postal survey of UK families. *Eur Child Adolesc Psychiatry*, **16**, 16–24.

Hancock E, O'Callaghan F, Osborne JP. (2005). Effect of melatonin dosage on sleep disorder in tuberous sclerosis complex. *J Child Neurol*, **20**, 78–80.

Hunt A. (1993). Development, behaviour and seizures in 300 cases of tuberous sclerosis. *J Intellect Disabil Res*, **37**, 41–51.

Hunt A, Stores G. (1994). Sleep disorder and epilepsy in children with tuberous sclerosis: a questionnaire-based study. *Dev Med Child Neurol*, **36**, 108–15.

Prather P, de Vries PJ. (2004). Behavioral and cognitive aspects of tuberous sclerosis complex. *J Child Neurol*, **19**, 666–74.

Thiele EA. (2004). Managing epilepsy in tuberous sclerosis complex. *J Child Neurol*, **19**, 680–6.

van Eeghen AM, Numis AI, Staley BA *et al.* (2011). Characterizing sleep disorders of adults with tuberous sclerosis complex: a questionnaire-based study and review. *Epilepsy Behav*, **20**, 68–74.

Wiznitzer M. (2004). Autism and tuberous sclerosis. *J Child Neurol*, **19**, 675–9.

Neurofibromatosis type 1 (NF-1)

Of the two types of neurofibromatosis, type 1 is the most common with a potentially complex and highly variable phenotype which includes the formation of tumours on nerve tissues throughout the body, café au lait spots, scoliosis, eye problems, epilepsy, intellectual impairment, and behavioural and psychiatric problems. Although an autosomal dominant condition, in 50% of cases it is the result of a spontaneous mutation. The abnormal gene is located at 17q11.2 (NF-1). NF-1 occurs in about 1 in 3000 births.

Sleep disturbance

Parents of children with NF-1have consistently complained that their children's sleep is often disturbed (Wadsby *et al.*, 1989; Samuelsson & Riccardi, 1989; Johnson *et al.*, 2005; Licis *et al.*, 2013). Leschziner *et al.* (2013) described sleep disturbance as part of the NF-1 phenotype in adults.

Types of sleep disturbance

In addition to the likely behavioural origin of such sleep problems, Johnson *et al.* (2005) described sleepwalking and sleep terrors. Licis *et al.* (2013) reported that, compared with their unaffected siblings, according to their parents children with NF-1 had significantly more settling and night waking problems, sleep–wake transition disorders such as rhythmic movements, vivid dreams, leg jerking while asleep, sleep-talking, and bruxism, and disorders of arousal including sleep-walking, night terrors and nightmares. In their adult series, Leschziner *et al.* (2013) found high rates of difficulty getting to sleep, waking in the night and early morning waking, as well as excessive daytime sleepiness with features suggestive of periodic limb movements, sleep disordered breathing and confusion on waking possibly caused by nocturnal seizures or other parasomnias. Specific respiratory factors have occasionally been described in some patients e.g. sleep apnoea associated with superior vena cava obstruction (Stradling *et al.*, 1981) and central alveolar hypoventilation syndrome, possibly the result of brain stem lesions (Sforza *et al.*, 1994).

Factors potentially contributing to sleep disturbance

Leschziner *et al.* (2013) have considered the many factors that might contribute to sleep disturbance in adults with NF-1. Further investigation might show how far the same considerations apply to children with the same condition. Possible examples are as follows.

Pathophysiological. Possibilities of this type include lesions in the brainstem affecting sleep architecture or REM sleep, those affecting the upper airway causing sleep disordered breathing, spinal cord compression producing spasticity, bladder dysfunction causing sleep fragmentation, peripheral neuropathy predisposing to restless legs syndrome or periodic limb movement disorder, and pain or discomfort or its treatment (such as tricyclic antidepressants for neuropathic pain which can reduce sleep quality or provoke periodic limb movement disorder). Intellectual impairment and other deficiencies in the cognitive profile of NF-1 are described (Levine *et al.*, 2006)

Physical comorbidities. The diversity of possible comorbidities of this type can be seen from the various pathophysiological factors just mentioned. In addition, epilepsy and some of its treatments may cause insomnia or excessive sleepiness.

Psychiatric comorbidities. Psychiatric disorders, especially depression and anxiety, and their pharmacological treatment, were also mentioned by Leschziner *et al.* (2013). In the case of children, to this last possibility can be added various behavioural problems including conduct disorder (Johnson *et al.*, 2005) and attention deficit hyperactivity disorder (Mautner *et al.*, 2002). Autism spectrum disorder has also been reported (Walsh *et al.*, 2013).

Medication effects are to be considered especially in children with the additional complications of the condition as mentioned above.

Parenting. Considering the potential complexity of their child's condition and its possible consequences for his social and emotional functioning (Martin *et al.*, 2012), it is no surprise that parents' responses to the diagnosis of NF-1 can be so distressing and likely to affect their parenting abilities (Ablon, 2000).

Aspects of assessment and management of the sleep disturbance

In addition to the general principles stated in Chapter 1, both assessment and treatment may need to match this complicated possible aetiology of sleep disturbance in NF-1.

Ablon J. (2000). Parents' responses to their child's diagnosis of neurofibromatosis 1. *Am J Med Genet*, **93**, 136–42.

Johnson H, Wiggs L, Stores G, Huson SM. (2005). Psychological disturbance and sleep disorders in children with neurofibromatosis type 1. *Dev Men Child Neurol*, **47**, 237–42.

Leschziner GD, Golding JF, Ferner RE. (2013). Sleep disturbance as part of the neurofibromatosis type 1 phenotype in adults. *Am J Med Genet A*, **161A**, 1319–22.

Levine TM, Materek A, Abel J, O'Donnell M, Cutting LE. (2006). Cognitive profile of neurofibromatosis type 1. *Semin Pediatr Neurol*, **13**, 8–20.

Licis AK, Vallorani A, Gao F *et al.* (2013). Prevalence of sleep disturbances in children with neurofibromatosis type 1. *J Child Neurol*, **28**, 1400–5.

Martin S, Wolters P, Baldwin A *et al.* (2012). Social-emotional functioning of children and adolescents with neurofibromatosis type 1 and plexiform neurofibromas: relationships with cognitive, disease, and environmental variables. *J Pediatr Psychol*, **37**, 713–24.

Mautner VF, Kluwe L, Thakker SD, Leark RA. (2002). Treatment of ADHD in neurofibromatosis type 1. *Dev Med Child Neurol*, **44**, 164–70.

Samuelsson B, Riccardi VM. (1989). Neurofibromatosis in Gothenberg, Sweden. III. Psychiatric and social aspects. *Neurofibromatosis*, **2**, 84–106.

Sforza E, Colamaria V, Lugaresi E. (1994). Neurofibromatosis associated with central alveolar hypoventilation syndrome during sleep. *Acta Paediatr*, **83**, 794–6.

Stradling JR, Huddart S, Arnold AG. (1981). Sleep apnoea syndrome caused by neuro-fibromatosis and superior vena caval obstruction. *Thorax*, **36**, 634–5.

Wadsby M, Lindehammar H, Eeg-Olofsson O. (1989). Neurofibromatosis in childhood: neuropsychological aspects. *Neurofibromatosis*, **2**, 251–60.

Walsh KS, Vélez JI, Kardel PG *et al.* (2013). Symptomatology of autism spectrum disorder in a population with neurofibromatosis type 1. *Dev Med Child Neurol*, **55**, 131–8.

Williams syndrome (WS)

This neurodevelopmental disorder is caused by a microdeletion of many genes on chromosome 7q11.23 which results in a complex phenotype with medical, cognitive and behavioural components. The characteristic dysmorphic facial appearance in childhood (sometimes referred to as 'elfin' or 'pixie-like') includes a short, upturned nose, wide mouth, full lips and cheeks, peri-orbital fullness, broad forehead and small jaw. Individuals have high levels of non-social anxiety and fears despite being very sociable and indeed over-friendly. The prevalence of WS is approximately 1 in 7500 individuals.

Occurrence of sleep disturbance
The few sleep studies on children with WS indicate a high rate of sleep disturbance. In a questionnaire study by Annaz *et al.* (2011), 97% of parents reported that their children with WS had sleep problems.

Types of sleep disturbance
The usual insomnia problems of settling and night waking difficulties appear to be commonplace in WS (Einfield *et al.*, 1997). Arens *et al.* (1998) reported restless sleep and prominent periodic limb movements which might account for the daytime sleepiness reported by Goldman *et al.* (2009) in children and adolescents with WS despite apparently normal amount of overnight sleep. In this report, restless legs syndrome and sleep apnoea were also mentioned as possible contributory factors.

The sleep problems reported by Annaz *et al.* (2011) took the form of bedtime resistance and delay in going to sleep, sleep anxiety, night waking, daytime sleepiness and nocturnal enuresis. Despite habitual snoring being quite common, there was no particular suggestion of OSA, or associations with various reported medical conditions. The study of children with WS by Mason *et al.* (2011), which included overnight polysomnography as well as a parental sleep questionnaire, also demonstrated a high prevalence of sleep disturbance and also attention deficit hyperactivity disorder-type symptoms but without any clear association between the two. Ashworth *et al.* (2013) reported that, compared with those with Down syndrome, children with WS had higher rates of bedtime problems and bedwetting.

Factors potentially contributing to sleep disturbance
Physical comorbidities. Widespread medical problems capable of disturbing sleep can occur in WS (Pober, 2010). These can take the form of cardiovascular, endocrine, gastrointestinal or neurological complications and overall cognitive impairment.

Psychiatric comorbidities. The anxiety, fears and phobias in WS described by Dykens (2003) and the attention deficit hyperactivity disorder-type behaviours emphasized in the findings of Leyfer *et al.* (2006) and Mason *et al.* (2011) appear to be common. Other findings in the study by Leyfer *et al.* (2006) were frequent descriptions by parents of specific phobias (especially of loud noises) and generalized anxiety states. Overall, psychiatric disorder was described in 78% of the children.

Other factors. Intrinsic pathophysiological processes likely to affect sleep have not been identified. Possible parenting and medication effects need to be considered in assessment and treatment as in other neurodevelopmental disorders. Axelsson *et al.* (2013) found more reports by mothers of sleeplessness in their toddlers with WS compared with typically developing children. This was associated with mothers' own poor quality sleep and mood change, as well as the affected children's level of language development.

Sleep assessment
The same principles apply as in other neurodevelopmental disorders.

Aspects of management of the sleep disturbance
In the current absence of information in the literature about treatments for sleep disturbance specifically in children with WS, general principles apply. Regarding the treatment of comorbid psychiatric conditions in children with WS, Green *et al.* (2012) report a high success rate with the use of stimulants for attention deficit hyperactivity disorder symptoms, and Pober (2010) refers to adolescents and adults being treated with an anxiolytic agent and other patients with antipsychotic medication but to what real effect is unclear.

Annaz D, Hill CM, Ashworth A, Holley S, Karmiloff-Smith A. (2011). Characterisation of sleep problems in children with Williams syndrome. *Res Dev Disabil*, **32**, 164–9.

Arens R, Wright B, Elliott J *et al.* (1998). Periodic limb movement in sleep in children with Williams syndrome. *J Pediatr*, **133**, 670–4.

Ashworth A, Hill CM, Karmiloff-Smith A, Dimitriou D. (2013). Cross syndrome comparison of sleep problems in children with Down syndrome and Williams syndrome. *Res Dev Disabil*, **34**, 1572–80.

Axelsson EL, Hill CM, Sadeh A, Dimitriou D. (2013). Sleep problems and language development in toddlers with Williams syndrome. *Res Dev Disabil*, **34**, 3988–96.

Dykens EM. (2003). Anxiety, fears, and phobias in persons with Williams syndrome. *Dev Neuropsychol*, **23**, 291–316.

Einfeld SL, Tonge BJ, Florio T. (1997). Behavioral and emotional disturbance in individuals with Williams syndrome. *Am J Ment Retard*, **102**, 45–53.

Goldman SE, Malow BA, Newman KD, Roof E, Dykens EM. (2009). Sleep patterns and daytime sleepiness in adolescents and young adults with Williams syndrome. *J Intellect Disabil Res*, **53**, 182–8.

Green T, Avda S, Dotan I *et al.* (2012). Phenotypic psychiatric characterization of children with Williams syndrome and response of those with ADHD to methylphenidate treatment. *Am J Med Genet B Neuropsychiatr Genet*, **159B**, 13–20.

Leyfer OT, Woodruff-Borden J, Klein-Tasman BP, Fricke JS, Mervis CB. (2006). Prevalence of psychiatric disorders in 4 to 16-year-olds with Williams syndrome. *Am J Med Genet B Neuropsychiatr Genet*, **141B**, 615–22.

Mason TB, Arens R, Sharman J *et al.* (2011). Sleep in children with Williams Syndrome. *Sleep Med*, **12**, 892–7.

Pober BR. (2010). Williams–Beuren syndrome. *N Engl J Med*, **362**, 239–52.

Deafblindness syndromes

As discussed in Chapter 3, comorbid visual or hearing impairment can contribute significantly to sleep disturbance. A combination of the two ('deafblindness' or 'dual sensory impairment'), of which there are congenital and acquired causes, can be expected to intensify this effect.

CHARGE syndrome (Blake & Prasad, 2006) is a main cause of congenital deafblindness. Of the children in the Denmark survey of the many causes of deafblindness reported by Dammeyer (2012), the largest group (16%) had a diagnosis of CHARGE syndrome.

The name is based on the following defects originally identified in children with the syndrome:

C: Coloboma of the eye
H: Heart defects
A: Atresia of the choanae
R: Retardation of growth and/or development
G: Genital and/or urinary defects (especially cryptorchidism and hypospadias)
E: Ear anomalies and deafness

However, these abnormalities alone are no longer used for formal diagnosis which rests on a combination of some of these features and many other possible congenital anomalies, as well as genetic testing which usually indicates an autosomal dominant disorder involving mutations on the CHD7 gene located on chromosome 8. The syndrome is reported to occur in about 1 in 10,000 live births.

Aspects of the sleep disturbance

Hartshorne *et al.* (2009) reported that nearly 60% of their series of children with CHARGE syndrome had significant sleep problems mainly taking the form of settling to sleep, staying asleep and sleep related breathing problems, which were associated with high caregiver malaise scores. Trider *et al.* (2012) also described high rates of sleep disturbance in their series including, in a high proportion, features of obstructive sleep apnoea (assessed by means of parental questionnaire) which responded to conventional treatment although this was followed by residual symptoms affecting the children's quality of life. In their assessment of various aspects of UK children with a diagnosis of CHARGE syndrome, Deuce *et al.* (2012) included sleep difficulties as a problem reported by parents, for which many of the children were taking regular medication (details not provided).

Principal causes of sleep disturbance in deafblind children in general are the sensory deficits themselves (see Chapter 3 for visual and hearing deficits considered separately), the effects of which are likely to be made worse when combined. However, possible additional influences may well contribute to sleep problems. In the case of CHARGE syndrome, these include intellectual impairment of various degrees (which Sanlaville and Verloes (2007) suggest might be the result of a combination of primary neurodevelopmental factors and acquired postnatal damages such as anoxo-ischaemic brain lesions) and various psychiatric and neuropsychiatric conditions, namely, obsessive-compulsive disorder, challenging behaviours (Blake & Pasad, 2006), attention deficit hyperactivity disorder, and Tourette syndrome (Hartshorne *et al.*, 2009).

Autism may also be diagnosed although it is suggested that this may well be over-diagnosed because of the difficulties of distinguishing between the features of primary autism spectrum disorder and behaviours caused by deafblindness itself, especially in the presence of intellectual impairment (Hoevenaars-van den Boom *et al.*, 2009). The same point was made by Graham *et al.* (2005) who reported that autism spectrum disorder-like behaviour (social withdrawal, lack of interest in social contact, hyperactivity and a need to maintain order) was more associated with CHARGE syndrome rather than with Down syndrome, Prader–Willi syndrome or Williams syndrome. As in other neurodevelopmental disorders, the effects of parenting stress in raising a child with CHARGE syndrome (Wulffaert *et al.*, 2009) – and other causes of deafblindness – is likely to interfere with the ability to encourage satisfactory sleep patterns in their child. All of these possible aetiological factors have to be taken into account in assessment and treatment including help and support for families in view of the stress that the disorder imposes (Wulffaert *et al.*, 2009).

Usher syndrome, another leading cause of deafblindness, is characterized by sensorineural deafness, associated with a defective inner ear, and gradual loss of vision caused by retinitis pigmentosa. Three clinical subtypes are described. Children with type I are born profoundly deaf, begin to lose their vision in the first decade and have gait and balance difficulties because of their defective vestibular system. Those with type II have hearing loss but are not profoundly deaf. Starting in their second decade, they begin to lose their vision. Balance problems are not a feature. In type III, children are also not deaf when born but afterwards have a gradual loss of their hearing and vision, and may have difficulties with balance. Usher syndrome is inherited as an autosomal recessive condition. It is associated with a mutation in any one of a number of genes on different loci resulting in a combination of hearing loss and visual impairment.

Aspects of the sleep disturbance

Sleep disturbance in Usher syndrome has been little studied. Dammeyer (2012) compared the development and clinical characteristics of children with the syndrome and others with CHARGE syndrome. Frequent sleep problems (nature unspecified) were reported in approximately 50% of both groups. Lesser degrees of severity were also about equal. The potential contributory factors in Usher syndrome to which reference is made in the same article are intellectual impairment which tends to be more pronounced in CHARGE syndrome, and (often based on single case studies) psychiatric disorders such as attention deficit hyperactivity disorder and psychosis. As usual, parental factors are also likely to be relevant. Clearly, much needs to be done to clarify the nature and causes of sleep disturbance in children with Usher syndrome as well as appropriate treatment procedures.

Blake KD, Prasad C. (2006). CHARGE syndrome. *Orphanet J Rare Dis*, **1**, 34.

Dammeyer J. (2012). Development and characteristics of children with Usher syndrome and CHARGE syndrome. *Int J Pediatr Otorhinolaryngol*, **76**, 1292–6.

Deuce G, Howard GS, Rose S, Fuggle C. (2012). A study of CHARGE syndrome in the UK. *Brit J Vis Impair*, **30**, 91–100.

Graham JM, Rosner B, Dykens E, Visootsak J. (2005). Behavioral features of CHARGE syndrome (Hall–Hittner syndrome) comparison with Down syndrome, Prader–Willi syndrome, and Williams syndrome. *Am J Med Genet A*, **133A**, 240–7.

Hartshorne TS, Heussler HS, Dailor AN *et al.* (2009). Sleep disturbances in CHARGE syndrome: types and relationships with behavior and caregiver well-being. *Dev Med Child Neurol*, **51**, 143–50.

Hoevenaars-van den Boom MA, Antonissen AC, Knoors H, Vervloed MP. (2009). Differentiating characteristics of deafblindness and autism in people with congenital deafblindness and profound intellectual disability. *J Intellect Disabil Res*, **53**, 548–58.

Sanlaville D, Verloes A. (2007). CHARGE syndrome: an update. *Eur J Hum Genet*, **15**, 389–99.

Trider CL, Corsten G, Morrison D *et al.* (2012). Understanding obstructive sleep apnea in children with CHARGE syndrome. *Int J Pediatr Otorhinolaryngol*, **76**, 947–53.

Wulffaert J, Scholte EM, Dijkxhoorn YM *et al.* (2009). Parenting stress in CHARGE syndrome and the relationship with child characteristics. *J Dev Phys Disabil*, **21**, 301–13.

Craniofacial syndromes

The craniofacial dysostosis syndromes are a group of inherited, congenital anomalies which cause abnormalities of the cranium, orbit and mid-face and sometimes the limbs. The more common of these syndromes include Apert, Crouzon and Pfeiffer syndromes. These syndromes are caused by mutations and almost all are inherited in an autosomal dominant fashion, the fibroblast growth factor receptor genes being primarily affected. An important issue is the potential for increased pressure on the brain with consequent problems with neural development, including visual problems. Mid-face deformities can be severe. Intellectual impairment varies widely.

Aspects of the sleep disturbance

Discussion of abnormal sleep in these syndromes has largely been confined to sleep disordered breathing caused by typical anatomical malformations as well as physiological dysfunction (Ali-Dinar & Ferraro, 2011). In addition to craniosynostosis predisposing to OSA and central apnoea, hypoventilation in sleep, obstructive sleep apnoea and central sleep apnoea can be the result of mandibular hypoplasia in Pierre Robin and Treacher Collins syndromes, skeletal disorder in achondroplasia, and the anatomical abnormalities in Arnold–Chiari malformation and Down syndrome (Simakajornboom & Beckerman, 2001). The importance of objective sleep studies for the identification of OSA is stressed by some authors such as Akre *et al.* (2012) in respect of Treacher Collins syndrome.

In discussing the management of such disorders, the last-mentioned authors make the point that attention needs to be paid not only to the sleep disorders of physiological origin, such as OSA for which regular screening was stressed by Pijpers *et al.* (2004), but also those of a behavioural nature as can be expected in many cases. Unfortunately there seems to be little or no study of this aspect despite the evidence that the quality of life of both children with craniofacial disorders and their parents suffers significantly (Bannink *et al.*, 2010; Roberts & Shute, 2011; de Jong *et al.*, 2012) in a way that can be expected to cause family and other psychosocial difficulties.

Akre H, Øverland B, Åsten P, Skogedal N, Heimdal K. (2012). Obstructive sleep apnea in Treacher Collins syndrome. *Eur Arch Otorhinolaryngol*, **212**, 269, 331–7.

Ali-Dinar T, Ferraro NF. Craniofacial disorders and sleep. In: Kothare SV, Kotagal S, eds. *Sleep in Childhood Neurological Disorders*. New York: demos Medical 2011. 387–97.

Bannink N, Maliepaard M, Raat H, Joosten KF, Mathijssen IM. (2010). Health-related quality of life in children and adolescents with syndromic craniosynostosis. *J Plast Reconstr Aesthet Surg*, **63**, 1972–81.

de Jong T, Maliepaard M, Bannink N, Raat H, Mathijssen IM. (2012). Health-related problems and quality of life in patients with syndromic and complex craniosynostosis. *Childs Nerv Syst*, **28**, 879–82.

Pijpers M, Poels PJ, Vaandrager JM *et al.* (2004). Undiagnosed obstructive sleep apnea syndrome in children with syndromal craniofacial synostosis. *J Craniofac Surg*, **15**, 670–4.

Roberts RM, Shute R. (2011). Children's experience of living with craniofacial condition: perspectives of children and parents. *Clin Child Psychol Psychiatry*, **16**, 317–34.

Simakajornboon N, Beckerman R. Sleep disorders and craniofacial syndromes. In: Stores G, Wiggs L, eds. *Sleep Disturbance in Children and Adolescents with Disorders of Development: its Significance and Management*. Clinics in Developmental Medicine No. 155. London: Mac Keith Press 2001. 64–72.

Neuromuscular disease

The term 'neuromuscular disease' refers to a broad category of conditions in which there is impairment of muscle function because of muscle pathology or pathology of nerves or neuromuscular junctions. Neuromuscular diseases may be acquired as in poliomyelitis, for example, but the most common are genetic in origin, e.g. Duchenne muscular dystrophy. Specific genes have been identified for over 100 neuromuscular diseases. Commonly symptoms of neuromuscular disease include infantile floppiness or hypotonia, delay in motor milestones, feeding and respiratory difficulties, abnormal gait characteristics, frequent falls, difficulty with stairs or arising from the floor, and muscle cramps or stiffness.

Aspects of the sleep disturbance

Although not the only type of sleep disturbance reported in children with neuromuscular disease, much of the literature has been concerned with sleep disordered breathing, especially OSA, but also central sleep apnoea and nocturnal hypoventilation. As in other children with sleep disordered breathing, complications can include cardiovascular and metabolic disease, and also cognitive and behavioural problems (see Chapter 1). Katz and D'Ambrosio (2011) have discussed the management of sleep disordered breathing in a wide range of childhood conditions which involve neuromuscular disease including Rett syndrome, Prader–Willi syndrome, cerebral palsy, Down syndrome, Duchenne muscular dystrophy and spinal muscular atrophy.

Bloetzer et al. (2012) reported a much higher prevalence of sleep disturbance in children with Duchenne muscular dystrophy compared with children in general. Main types of sleep problem included difficulty settling to sleep or staying asleep at night, sleep related breathing disorder and excessive daytime sleepiness, discomfort at night, steroid treatment (known to affect behaviour), and single-parent household (possibly subject to increased psychosocial stress). Arguing that Duchenne muscular dystrophy is not only a muscular disorder but also a disorder affecting the brain, Hendriksen & Vles (2008) reported associations between it and attention deficit hyperactivity disorder, autism spectrum disorder and obsessive-compulsive disorder (all linked with sleep disturbances, as described elsewhere in this chapter).

Martinez-Rodriguez (2010) described excessive daytime sleepiness as a prominent complaint in myotonic dystrophy type 1, the classical and congenital forms of which occur in childhood (although the author makes the point that early detection is rare because clinicians tend to pay little attention to sleepiness when taking a medical history). Also, excessive daytime sleepiness is often misinterpreted. Its degree can be severe consisting (like narcolepsy) of continuous excessive sleepiness during the day as well as sleep attacks. This sleepiness (which is distinct from the common accompanying complaint of fatigue) is not simply attributable to sleep disordered breathing and is thought more likely to be caused by an intrinsic central nervous system dysfunction affecting systems controlling the sleep–wake cycle. Both amphetamine-like stimulants and modafinil are said to have been used to good effect if sleep disordered breathing is not present or has failed to respond to the usual treatments (Laberge et al., 2013).

Parenting factors (and other behavioural issues likely to contribute to sleep disturbance in children with neuromuscular disease) seem to have received little attention, although Hemmingsson.et al. (2009) have emphasized the association between sleep problems and the need of children with physical disabilities for attention from their parents at night. This may include the need to reposition them in bed because of their inability to change position to avoid pain or discomfort.

Bloetzer C, Jeannet PY, Lynch B, Newman CJ. (2012). Sleep disorders in boys with Duchenne muscular dystrophy. *Acta Paediatr*, **101**, 1265–9.

Hemmingsson H, Stenhammar AM, Paulsson K. (2009). Sleep problems and the need for parental night-time attention in children with physical disabilities. *Child Care Health Dev*, **35**, 89–95.

Hendriksen JG, Vles JS. (2008). Neuropsychiatric disorders in males with duchenne muscular dystrophy: frequency rate of attention deficit hyperactivity disorder (ADHD), autism spectrum disorder, and obsessive-compulsive disorder. *J Child Neurol*, **23**, 477–81.

Katz ES, D'Ambrosio CM. Management of sleep disordered breathing in children with neuromuscular disease. In: Kothare SV, Kotagal S, eds. *Sleep in Childhood Neurological Disorders*. New York: demos Medical 2011. 275–94.

Laberge L, Gagnon C, Dauvilliers Y. (2013). Daytime sleepiness and myotonic dystrophy. *Curr Neurol Neurosci Rep*, **13**, 340.

Martinez-Rodriguez JE. Myotonic dystrophy. In: Overeem S, Reading P, eds. *Sleep Disorders in Neurology, a Practical Approach*. Oxford: Wiley-Blackwell 2010. 139–46.

Cornelia de Lange syndrome (CdLS)

This rare condition, due to genetic mutations on chromosomes 5p13, Xp11 and 10q25, is characterized by many abnormalities including dysmorphic facial features, delayed growth, various degrees of intellectual impairment, and malformations of the musculoskeletal and other systems. It occurs in 1 in 10,000–50,000 births.

Aspects of the sleep disturbance

Sleep problems have been reported as commonplace in children and adults with CdLS (Berney *et al.*, 1999; Hall *et al.*, 2008; Rajan *et al.*, 2012). The last study emphasized insomnia, especially in children, with the possibility of a circadian rhythm disorder. Stavinoha *et al.* (2011) have reported that sleep disordered breathing and sleepiness appear to be common, but the nature of specific under-lying sleep disorders has not been established in any detail. There are many potential sleep disturbing factors to consider, including the various physical health problems discussed by Hall *et al.* (2008), such as epilepsy and gastro-oesophageal reflux. Likewise, a variety of psychiatric problems have been reported by Berney *et al.* (1999) and Basile *et al.* (2007), namely hyperactivity, attention disorder, anxiety and compulsive disorder, aggression, self-injurious behaviour and an autism-like syndrome, as well as intellectual impairment. Moss *et al.* (2008) have also reported autism spectrum disorder in over two-thirds of their series of children with CdLS. The implications for assessment and management of this complexity are clear.

Basile E, Villa L, Selicorni A, Molteni M. (2007). The behavioural phenotype of Cornelia de Lange syndrome: a study of 56 individuals. *J Intellect Disabil Res*, **51**, 671–81.

Berney TP, Ireland M, Burn J. (1999). Behavioural phenotype of Cornelia de Lange syndrome. *Arch Dis Child*, **81**, 333–6.

Hall SS, Arron K, Sloneem J, Oliver C. (2008). Health and sleep problems in Cornelia de Lange Syndrome: a case control study. *J Intellect Disabil Res*, **52**, 458–68.

Moss JF, Oliver C, Berg K. (2008). Prevalence of autistic spectrum phenomenology in Cornelia de Lange and Cri du Chat syndromes. *Am J Ment Retard*, **113**, 278–91.

Rajan R, Benke JR, Kline AD. (2012). Insomnia in Cornelia de Lange syndrome. *Int J Pediatr Otorhinolaryngol*, **76**, 972–5.

Stavinoha RC, Kline AD, Levy HP *et al.* (2011). Characterisation of sleep disturbance in Cornelia de Lange syndrome. *Int J Pediatr Otorhinolaryngol*, **75**, 215–18.

Cri du Chat syndrome (CDC)

This condition, which occurs in 1 in 50,000 live births, is caused by a partial deletion in the short arm of chromosome 5. Its many possible characteristics include a cat-like cry, low birth weight, early feeding difficulties, abnormalities of the face and head, congenital scoliosis, gastro-intestinal and cardiovascular problems, and intellectual impairment.

Aspects of the sleep disturbance

This seems to be a significant problem in many children with CDC. For example, Cornish *et al.* (1996) reported that it was a serious concern to nearly half of the parents in their sample, especially in the form of night awakenings but also settling problems. The latter finding, however, was not confirmed by Maas *et al.* (2009) but in their study based on a parental sleep questionnaire the following additional types of sleep disturbance were prominent in the CDC group: poor quality sleep (judged in terms of restless sleep and excessive daytime sleepiness), headbanging during sleep or when going off to sleep, anxieties about sleep (e.g. needing a security object and enacting bedtime rituals), and disordered breathing during sleep, especially snoring, although not usually associated with apnoeas.

This study was followed by a comparison of sleep disturbance in children and adults with CDC, Down syndrome, Jacobsen syndrome (see later) and a mixed group of children with intellectual impairment (Maas *et al.*, 2012). Main findings were that sleep problems were not more common in the three syndrome groups than in the mixed group of patients, that in all three of the syndrome groups snoring (without other symptoms to suggest sleep apnoea) was the most prevalent type of sleep disturbance, and that complaints about sleep by parents or other caregivers were particularly common in the Jacobsen syndrome group.

The aetiology of these types of sleep disturbance in the individual child needs to be considered. In CDC this will include consideration of the varied degree of intellectual impairment (usually in the moderate to severe range), comorbid medical problems of which many possibilities are mentioned in the sample studied by Maas *et al.* (2009) such as epilepsy and upper respiratory tract infections, and a range of reported behaviour problems associated with CDC to which the authors refer. These include self-injury, sensory hypersensitivity, obsessional behaviour, hyperactivity, attention problems, aggression, and temper tantrums. Autistic features were mentioned by Dykens and Clarke (1997), and Moss *et al.* (2008) reported autism spectrum disorder in over a third of their series. As little of note has been published about the value of specific treatments in patients with CDC, it is appropriate to apply the general management principles described in earlier chapters.

Cornish KM, Pigram J. (1996). Developmental and behavioural characteristics of Cri du Chat syndrome. *Arch Dis Child*, **75**, 448–50.

Dykens EM, Clarke DJ. (1997). Correlates of maladaptive behavior in individuals with 5p- (Cri du Chat) syndrome. *Dev Med Child Neurol*, **39**, 752–6.

Maas APHM, Didden R, Korzilius H et al. (2009). Sleep in individuals with Cri du Chat syndrome: a comparative study. *J Intell Disabil Res*, **53**, 704–15

Maas APHM, Didden R, Korzilius H, Curfs LMG. (2012). Exploration of differences in types of sleep disturbance and severity of sleep problems between individuals with Cri du Chat syndrome, Down's syndrome and Jacobsen syndrome: a case control study. *Res Dev Dis*, **33**, 1773–9.

Moss JF, Oliver C, Berg K. (2008). Prevalence of autistic spectrum phenomenology in Cornelia de Lange and Cri du Chat syndromes. *Am J Ment Retard*, **113**, 278–91.

Juvenile neuronal ceroid-lipofuscinosis (JNCL)

Neuronal ceroid lipofuscinosis (NCL) refers to a group of neurodegenerative diseases, the various forms of which include infantile NCL (INCL), late-infantile NCL (LINCL), and juvenile NCL (JNCL). The term Batten disease was once regarded as the juvenile form of NCL but it is often used to describe all forms of NCL. These subtypes differ from each other regarding age of onset and progression of their condition. JNCL is the most prevalent form in which ceroid and lipofuscin material accumulates in body tissues including the CNS, causing progressive loss of vision, intellectual deterioration, gradually worsening epilepsy and other defects affecting various systems. It is inherited as an autosomal recessive condition due to mutation at the CLN3 gene on chromosome16p12. Prevalence is estimated as 1 in 100,000 live births

Aspects of the sleep disturbance

Sleep problems have been reported to affect the majority of children with JNCL, mainly taking the form of settling problems, night-time awakenings and nightmares (Santavuori et al., 1993). Heikkilä et al. (1995) added sleep terrors and also sleep–wake cycle irregularities. Disturbed respiratory patterns during sleep (increasing with duration of the disease) were also described by Telakivi et al. (1985) but without sleep apnoea. Kirveskari et al. (2000) reported PSG findings in children with JNCL: many aspects of sleep architecture were different from that of healthy control children, together with paroxysmal epileptiform activity. The overall picture presented was that of a progressive complex disruption of sleep structure compatible with the various reported sleep complaints including excessive daytime sleepiness resulting from impaired sleep quality. Members of the same group described actometry evidence (thought to be the result of the circadian timing system) of excessive daytime sleepiness and abnormal circadian sleep–wake rhythms in a variant form of LINC (Kirveskari et al., 2001).

As usual in the neurodevelopmental disorders, the origins of the sleep disturbances in JNCL and treatment requirements are multifactorial. In addition to neuropathological factors, including intellectual impairment and epilepsy, influences of a psychiatric nature are highly likely. Such disturbances mentioned by Santavuori et al. (1993) included restlessness, anxiety, aggression, depression, and also hallucinations the nature of which was not specified.

Apparently, little has been written about management. A study of treatment for insomnia problems by Hätönen et al. (1999) involved three children with JNCL, one with INCL and another with LINCL. The findings suggested that melatonin was of limited value, especially in the last two patients who were in an advanced stage of their disease presumably to the extent that their circadian regulatory system was severely damaged and unresponsive to this form of treatment. Not least of all, when faced with their children's deteriorating condition, parents are likely to need much help and support to cope with the situation including their child's sleep disturbance.

Hätönen T, Kirveskari E, Heiskala H et al. (1999). Melatonin ineffective in neuronal ceroid lipofuscinosis patients with fragmented or normal motor activity rhythms recorded by wrist actigraphy. Mol Genet Meta, **66**, 401–6.

Heikkilä E, Hätönen TH, Telakivi T et al. (1995). Circadian rhythm studies in neuronal ceroid-lipofuscinosis (NCL). Am J Med Genet, **57**, 229–34.

Kirveskari E, Partinen M, Salmi T et al. (2000). Sleep alterations in juvenile neuronal ceroid-lipofuscinosis. Pediatr Neurol, **22**, 347–54.

Kirveskari E, Partinen M, Santavuori P. (2001). Sleep and its disturbance in a variant form of late infantile neuronal ceroid lipofuscinosis (CLN5). J Child Neurol, **16**, 707–13.

Santavuori P, Linnankivi T, Jaeken J et al. (1993). Psychological symptoms of sleep disturbances in neuronal ceroid-lipofuscinosis (NCL). Inherit Metab Dis, **16**, 245–8.

Telakivi T, Partinen M, Salmi T. (1985). Sleep disturbance in patients with juvenile neuronal ceroid-lipofuscinosis: a new application of the SCSB-method. J Ment Defic Res, **29** (Pt 1) 29–35.

Smith–Lemli–Opitz syndrome (SLOS)

This autosomal recessive metabolic disorder is caused by an abnormality in the production or synthesis of cholesterol due to a low occurrence of 7-DHC reductase, an enzyme involved in cholesterol synthesis. It is characterized by multiple congenital abnormalities including facial dysmorphism, growth deficiency, and varied degrees of intellectual impairment. SLOS occurs in 1:20,000–40,000 births.

Aspects of the sleep disturbance

Descriptions of the behavioural phenotype of SLOS commonly refer to sleep disturbance (Tierney et al., 2000; Diaz-Stransky & Tierney, 2012). From their questionnaire survey of sleep disturbance in children and adults with SLOS, Zarowski et al. (2011) reported frequent multiple sleep problems, i.e. insomnia (difficulty getting to sleep, troublesome night waking including needing their parents' company to fall asleep – presumably related to anxiety and disturbing sleep associations, and early morning waking), sleep disordered breathing, and excessive daytime sleepiness. In theory, such problems should be amenable to treatment. However, attention would also need to be paid to the mood disorder and attention deficit hyperactivity disorder described in SLOS by Diaz-Stransky and Tierney (2012) as well as the associated autism spectrum disorder emphasized by Sikora *et al.* (2006).

Diaz-Stransky A, Tierney E. (2012). Cognitive and behavioral aspects of Smith–Lemli–Opitz syndrome. *Am J Med Genet C Semin Med Genet*, **160C**, 295–300.

Sikora DM, Pettit-Kekel K, Penfield J, Merkens LS, Steiner RD. (2006). The near universal presence of autism spectrum disorders in children with Smith–Lemli–Opitz syndrome. *Am J Med Genet A*, **140**, 1511–18.

Tierney E, Nwokoro NA, Kelley RI. (2000). Behavioral phenotype of RSH/ Smith–Lemli–Opitz syndrome. *Ment Retard Dev Disabil Res Rev*, **6**, 131–4.

Zarowski M, Vendrame M, Irons M, Kothare SV. (2011). Prevalence of sleep problems in Smith–Lemli–Opitz syndrome. *Am J Med Genet A*, **155A**, 1558–62.

Niemann–Pick disease type C

This rare condition is caused by mutations in the NP-C genes leading to accumulation of cholesterol and glycosphingolipids in the brain and other tissues. Various characteristic neurological signs develop at different ages starting in infancy.

Epilepsy is said to be common (Patterson *et al.*, 2012). An association between NP-C and narcolepsy-cataplexy was reported in children by Challamel *et al.* (1994). In a later study by the same group, in addition to PSG evidence of extensive disruptions of sleep architecture, features of narcolepsy-cataplexy were again seen including low cerebrospinal fluid hypocretin levels (Vancova *et al.*, 2003). It was suggested that the lysosomal storage abnormalities which characterize the disease might have affected hypocretin-containing cells in the hypothalamus. Some accounts have referred to gelastic cataplexy (sudden loss of muscle tone associated with laughter) and sleep inversion (sleepiness during the day and wakefulness at night).

Challamel MJ, Mazzola ME, Nevsimalova S. (1994). Narcolepsy in children. *Sleep*, **17** (8 Suppl), S17–20.

Patterson MC, Hendriksz CJ, Walterfang M. (2012). Recommendations for the diagnosis and management of Niemann–Pick disease type C: an update. *Mol Genet Metab*, **106**, 330–44.

Vancova J, Stepanova I, Jech R. (2003). Sleep disturbances and hypocretin deficiency in Niemann–Pick disease type C. *Sleep*, **26**, 427–30.

Norrie disease

This disorder is caused by mutations in the NDP gene and is inherited in an X-linked recessive pattern.

Parkes *et al.* (1999) referred to a wide variety of sleep disturbance in Norrie disease (as well as Prader–Willi syndrome and Moebius syndrome) including daytime sleepiness parasomnias and cataplexy. Many aspects of the condition predispose to sleep disturbance, including congenital blindness, progressive hearing loss and intellectual impairment. Smith *et al.* (2012) also refer to epilepsy and various psychiatric disorders, especially autism.

Parkes JD. (1999). Genetic factors in human sleep disorders with special reference to Norrie disease, Orader-Willi syndrome and Moebius syndrome. *J Sleep Res*, **8** Suppl 1, 14–22.
Smith SE, Mullen TE, Graham D, Sims KB, Rehm HL. (2012). Norrie disease: extraocular clinical manifestations in 56 patients. *Am J Med Genet A*, **158A**, 1909–17.

Lesch–Nyhan syndrome

Little has been published about sleep aspects of this rare X-linked recessive disorder in which there is a deficiency of the enzyme hypoxanthine-guanine phosphoribosyl transferase which leads to a build-up of uric acid. This can result in severe aggression, self-mutilation and gout. Severe self-injury especially of the fingers and mouth is a prominent feature but various signs of neurological dysfunction, as well as cognitive and behavioral disturbances are common. LNS affects about 1 in 380,000 live births. Sleep studies appear to be confined to just two small PSG investigations. Mizuno *et al.* (1979) described in various patients reduced time asleep, decreased REM density and self-mutilation in sleep. Saito *et al.* (1998) reported REM and NREM abnormalities, and severe OSA in one case with hypothyroidism.

Mizuno T, Ohta R, Kodama K *et al.* (1979). Self-mutilation and sleep stage in the Lesch–Nyhan syndrome. *Brain Dev*, **1**, 121–5.
Saito Y, Hanaoka S, Fukumisu M. (1998). Polysomnographic studies of Lesch–Nyhan syndrome. *Brain Dev*, **20**, 579–85.

Jacobsen syndrome

This rare congenital disorder results from deletion of a terminal region of chromosome 11. Maas *et al.* (2008) reported settling difficulties, restless sleep and sleeping in unusual positions, frequent night waking and early morning waking. Maas *et al.* (2012) described differences in types of sleep disturbance and severity of sleep problems between patients with Jacobsen syndrome, Cri du Chat syndrome or Down syndrome. Snoring was the most prevalent type of sleep disturbance in all three groups, and overall complaints about sleep were particularly high in the Jacobsen syndrome group.

Maas AP, Grossfeld PD, Didden R *et al.* (2008). Sleep problems in individuals with 11q terminal deletion disorder (Jacobsen syndrome). *Genet Couns*, **19**, 225–35.
Maas APHM, Didden R, Korzilius H, Curfs LMG. (2012). Exploration of differences in types of sleep disturbance and severity of sleep problems between individuals with Cri du Chat syndrome, Down's syndrome and Jacobsen syndrome: a case control study. *Res Dev Dis*, **33**, 1773–9.

Other syndromes

There have been limited reports of sleep disturbance in children with some other neurodevelopmental syndromes. Sleep related breathing disorders are mentioned in aspartylglucosaminuria (Lindblom *et al.*, 2006), Coffin–Lowry syndrome (Norgren, 2013), Ehlers–Danlos syndrome (Guilleminault *et al.*, 2013), Fabry disease (Duning *et al.*, 2009, who also emphasize excessive sleepiness), Joubert syndrome (Kamdar *et al.*, 2011), Rubenstein–Taybi syndrome (Zucconi *et al.*, 1993), and Wolf–Hirschorn syndrome (Curfs *et al.*, 1999). As in neurodevelopmental disorders in general, in these (and other) conditions more detailed enquiry is likely to reveal additional sleep disturbances, notably insomnia, as well as various influences on sleep including comorbidities.

Curfs LMG, Didden R, Sikkema SPE de Die-Smulders CEM. (1999). Management of sleeping problems in Wolf–Hirschorn syndrome: a case study. *Genet Counsel*, **10**, 345–50.

Duning T, Deppe M, Keller S *et al.* (2009). Excessive daytime sleepiness is a common symptom in Fabry disease. *Case Rep Neurol*, **1**, 33–40.

Guilleminault C, Primeau M, Chiu HY *et al.* (2013). Sleep-disordered breathing in Ehlers–Danlos syndrome: a genetic model of OSA. *Chest*, **144**, 1503–11.

Kamdar BB, Nandkumar, Krishnan V *et al.* (2011). Self-reported sleep and breathing disturbances in Joubert syndrome. *Pediatr Neurol*, **45**, 395–9.

Lindblom N, Kivinen S, Heiskala H, Laakso ML, Kaski M. (2006). Sleep disturbances in aspartylglucosaminuria (AGU): a questionnaire study *J Inherit Metab Dis*, **29**, 637–46.

Norgren A. (2013). Coffin–Lowry syndrome. *Swedish Information Centre for Rare Diseases*.

Zucconi M, Ferini-Strambi L, Erminio C, Pestalozza G, Smirne S. (1993). Obstructive sleep apnea in the Rubenstein–Taybi syndrome. *Respiration*, **60**, 127–32.

Neuropsychiatric disorders

As mentioned in the opening part of this book, childhood 'neuropsychiatric disorders' can be viewed as a subset of neurodevelopmental disorders, characteristically involving prominent psychiatric disturbance nevertheless arising from neurological dysfunction the precise nature of which, for the most part, is ill-defined as yet. Children with this type of disorder generally attend child psychiatric services rather than those providing investigation and treatment by developmental paediatricians or paediatric neurologists.

Autism spectrum disorder (ASD)

ASD refers to a group of neurodevelopmental disorders the incidence of which is reported to have been increasing in recent years, although this might be the result of increased awareness and discussion. A prevalence rate in UK primary school age children of 116 per 10,000 has been estimated. The genetics of ASD has yet to be clarified. ASD has been diagnosed in many neurodevelopmental disorders suggesting the possibility of common biological mechanisms.

Box 7 The wild boy of Aveyron

Jean Marc Gaspard Itard (1775–1838) was a French physician with a special interest in diseases of the ear and the education of deaf children. He is credited with providing an early description of autism.

As a medical student he encountered "the wild boy of Aveyron" whom he called Victor. At the age of about 12, Victor had been found in the woods where he was thought to have been living wild for perhaps 8 years or so. He was naked, without speech although he could hear, and behaving somewhat like a wild animal.

Itard spent some years attempting (with some degree of success) to educate Victor and teach him language and civilized behaviour. The methods he developed are considered still relevant to the education of developmentally delayed children.

Some believe that various aspects of Victor's behaviour correspond to autism although, of course, his early life and mysterious origins and survival in the woods were far removed from those of typical autistic children. What little is reported about Victor's sleep reflects his early way of life. Initially he slept rolled up in a ball anywhere (although later in a bed) and was easily woken with somewhat agitated dreams but sometimes with bursts of laughter.

Wolf S. (2004). The history of autism. *Eur Child Adolesc Psychiatry*, 13, 201–8.
Lane H. *The Wild Boy of Aveyron*. Cambridge MA: Harvard University Press 1979.

DSM-5 refers to ASD without any subdivisions and with Rett syndrome and childhood disintegrative disorder now excluded. Contrary to the earlier view that 'autism' was of psychological origin, this group of disorders is now known to be undoubtedly neurological in nature (Silver & Rapin, 2012) with a strong genetic influence and some evidence of disturbed structure and function in various brain systems (Santangelo & Tsatsanis, 2005). Diagnostic criteria in DSM-5 have been rearranged into impaired social communication/interaction, and restricted and repetitive behaviours, with diagnosis based on current symptoms or by history.

Generalizations about the sleep disorders of children with ASD as a whole are of limited validity in view of the heterogeneous nature of this group. In fact, the heterogeneity does not stop there as there are multiple possible causes of ASD (including genetic, brain damage or dysfunction) and a range of possible comorbid developmental, medical and psychiatric disorders (Reynolds & Malow, 2011). Consequently, as in other neurodevelopmental disorders, various factors might be contributing to an individual child's sleep disturbance, each requiring its own type of attention, as far as possible.

Occurrence of sleep disturbance
There are now many reports which consistently describe particularly high rates of significant sleep problems in most children with ASD (Johnson *et al.*, 2009; Cortesi

et al., 2010). Consistently, parent-reported sleep problems are described in two-thirds or more of children with ASD, regardless of age or IQ level, and often the problems persist (Richdale & Schreck, 2009). Sleep disturbances occur across all cognitive levels, more marked in children showing autistic regression who also show greater general disruption of their sleep (Giannotti *et al.*, 2011). A longitudinal study demonstrated the persistence from 30 months of age to adolescence of a reduction of sleep duration (Humphreys *et al.*, 2014).

Types of sleep disturbance in ASD

Many forms of sleep problem are reported in children with ASD (Richdale & Schreck, 2009). The most common highlighted by parents of children with ASD have been forms of insomnia, i.e. difficulty settling to sleep (including resistance to doing so), waking during the night, early morning waking (sometimes extremely early) and overall reduction in duration of sleep. Parent-reported settling difficulties are reported to be more common in children with autism compared not only with typically developing children but also those with Down syndrome and Prader–Willi syndrome (Cotton & Richdale, 2006). The findings by Krakowiak *et al.* (2008) emphasized night waking problems. Such periods awake at night might last 2–3 hours during which time the child may laugh, talk or play without any expression of discontent (Wiggs & Stores, 2004). Highly irregular sleep–wake cycles have been described which might account for some of these forms of insomnia (Glickman, 2009). Baker *et al.* (2013) have reported that, compared with typically developing adolescents, those with high-functioning ASD have more symptoms of insomnia associated with increased daytime sleepiness.

Additional forms of disturbed sleep, such as daytime sleepiness and OSA, are also sometimes mentioned (Richdale & Schreck, 2009). The nature of the sleep disorders may change as the children move through adolescence (Goldman *et al.*, 2011). Parasomnias have also been reported to be more frequent in ASD children than in other groups (Schreck & Mulick, 2000). However, the nature of these parasomnias is unclear from the information available. This last report referred to nightmares, 'disorientated awakening' and also bruxism. Screaming episodes at night are open to a number of interpretations including sleep terrors. A preliminary study by Ming *et al.* (2009) suggested a high prevalence of parasomnias in children with ASD, especially of the arousal disorder type. Distinguishing between the various forms of dramatic parasomnias is likely to be particularly difficult in children with ASD if only because of communication problems, although sleep behaviour disorder (involving acting out of dreams) has been claimed in some children with ASD (Thirumalai *et al.*, 2002).

Factors potentially contributing to sleep disturbance

Various factors (perhaps in combination) might underlie sleep problems in children with ASD (Richdale & Schreck, 2009).

Pathophysiological. The neurological nature of ASD was mentioned earlier but the neuropathological details (including those which might affect sleep–wake systems) have yet to be defined (Silver & Rapin, 2012). However, some reports suggest that intrinsic physiological factors are implicated. For example, subtle abnormalities of NREM sleep in the form of cyclic alternating pattern (CAP) (Parrino *et al.*, 2012) have been suggested in some children with ASD (Miano *et al.* 2007), and sleep–wake rhythm disorders have been linked with an abnormal pattern of melatonin production (Kulman *et al.* 2000). According to Hollway and Aman (2011), the various possible correlates of insomnia in children with ASD included intellectual disability which occurs to some extent in about half of such children although in less than a fifth to a moderate to severe degree (Charman *et al.*, 2011).

ASD is one of several neurodevelopmental disorders such as Angelman syndrome, foetal alcohol spectrum disorder and ADHD (see elsewhere in this chapter) in which 'sensory processing disorder' has been described. As described in connection with FASD, this is a controversial concept not recognized in DSM or ICD systems. However, its treatment has been recommended by some authors for various conditions including sleep disturbance (Wengel *et al.*, 2011).

Physical comorbidities. Neurological comorbidities are common in ASD and are associated with more clinical severity (Jeste, 2011). Epilepsy occurs in about a third of children with this condition (Malow, 2004) and, as discussed in Chapter 3, it can disrupt sleep in various ways. Maski *et al.* (2011) have emphasized the importance of recognizing this (and other comorbidities) in ASD because of their potential adverse effects on the child's cognition and behaviour to which can be added sleep. A preliminary study by Youssef *et al.* (2013) found significantly lower serum ferritin levels in children with ASD compared with controls. Within the ASD group, most reduced ferritin levels were associated with a higher rate of sleep fragmentation and periodic limb movements in sleep.

Psychiatric comorbidities. Disturbed sleep in children with ASD is associated with various behavioural problems (Joshi *et al.*, 2010) including worsening of autistic symptoms (Sikora *et al.*, 2012). Successful treatment of the sleep problem may improve daytime behaviour (Richdale, 2001).

Simonoff *et al.* (2008) reported frequent, often multiple and persistent psychiatric disorders in children with ASD, the most common diagnoses being social anxiety disorder, ADHD and oppositional defiant disorder. Somewhat similar findings were reported by Leyfer *et al.* (2006) and Skokauskas and Gallagher (2012). Such problems can persist into adolescence (Simonoff *et al.*, 2013). In a separate study of adolescents with ASD, severe mood changes were common and associated with maternal mental health problems (Simonoff *et al.*, 2012). Joshi *et al.* (2010) reported that the vast majority of children and adolescents with ASD referred to a paediatric psychopharmacology programme had multiple comorbid psychiatric disorders. Based on their detailed review of the literature, the conclusions reached by Hollway and Aman (2011) were that the main predictors of insomnia in children with ASD appear to be severity of their disorder, anxiety, and depression. Other possible correlates were said to include intellectual level, inattention and hyperactivity, various comorbid medical conditions including epilepsy, and medication effects. The relationship between ASD and attention deficit hyperactivity disorder has been considered in detail by Matson, *et al.* (2013).

Medication effects. Murray *et al.* (2013) surveyed the psychotropic medications prescribed for young patients with ASD. They included psychostimulants for attention deficit hyperactivity disorder and antipsychotics both of which are capable of disturbing sleep. Other potentially sleep-disturbing medications were discussed in Chapter 1.

Parenting. The intellectual limitation and communication difficulties shown by many children with ASD are likely to interfere with their parents' efforts to teach their child satisfactory sleep habits. Difficulties handling bedtime and night waking problems, such as inadequate limit-setting, will contribute significantly to their child's behavioural sleep disturbance. Inappropriate bedtime routines involving stereotypical and repetitive behaviours or rituals are likely to cause settling problems in particular.

Parental reports of their autistic children's sleep problems have been found to be associated with self-reports of stress (Goodlin-Jones *et al.*, 2008). This might at least partly explain why their own sleep suffers more than that of other parents (Lopez-Wagner *et al.*, 2008; Meltzer, 2008) with consequences for parenting ability and other aspects of family life. Being stressed and tired, they might find it particularly difficult to cope with their children's sleep disturbance.

Associated neurodevelopmental disorders. Zafeiriou *et al.* (2007) has reviewed the range of other neurodevelopmental disorders with which ASD is associated and which may need to be taken into account in explaining and treating sleep disturbance in children with ASD. As described in more detail earlier in this chapter, main examples associated with disturbed sleep of one type or another are fragile X syndrome, Down syndrome, neurofibromatosis type 1, Angelman syndrome, Prader–Willi syndrome and Tourette syndrome.

Sleep assessment

Malow *et al.* (2012) have described a 'practice pathway' for identifying and managing insomnia in children and adolescents with ASD. They emphasize the importance of screening for insomnia problems with a view to introducing treatment initially in the form of parent education and behavioural methods and medication in certain situations, followed by careful follow-up. The need for repeated assessment of children with a neurodevelopmental disorder, as a check on progress and possible changes in the child's overall condition and circumstances, was emphasized in Chapter 2.

Some investigators have used objective sleep assessment to supplement parental reports. Polysomnographic comparisons between ASD 'good sleepers' and 'poor sleepers' have been reported to validate parental reports of bedtime settling difficulties and length of time their child sleeps; otherwise sleep physiology of both groups was the same as typically developing children (Malow *et al.*, 2006). A more complicated picture has been described in a study which included polysomnographic assessment which in children with ASD showed some correspondence with parental reports but also subtle differences in both NREM and REM sleep compared with controls (Miano *et al.*, 2007). The clinical significance of these findings is uncertain.

Sleep patterns measured by actigraphy do not always differ between those ASD children with or without reported sleeplessness (Wiggs & Stores, 2004). This and the fact that improvement in insomnia with treatment, as claimed by parents, may not be accompanied by objective change (see below) raises the question of whether the beneficial treatment effect involved changes in parental attitudes rather than physiological factors. Alternatively, it has been suggested that traditional objective measures might be relatively insensitive to more subtle aspects of sleep physiology such as cyclic alternating pattern or CAP (mentioned earlier), alterations of which might correspond better with subjective reports (Parrino *et al.*, 2012).

Aspects of management of sleep disturbance

Given the range of possible sleep disorders in ASD and its many factors potentially affecting sleep (each requiring management in its own right), various treatments might well be required, quite possibly in combination (Reynolds & Malow, 2011). Miano and Ferri (2010) have reviewed the available options.

Vriend *et al.* (2011) have discussed the limited information on the relative efficacy of the various types of behavioural interventions for sleep problems in children with ASD, concluding that standard extinction and scheduled awakenings come out best. Johnson *et al.* (2013) also assessed the few randomized controlled trials of behaviour treatments for sleep problems in children with ASD. The results of their own preliminary study of this type (the scope of which was confined to insomnia problems with exclusion of children with apparent physiological, medical or psychiatric factors which might be contributing to the sleep disturbances) suggested that a behavioural parent-training programme was effective. Malow *et al.* (2014) found that relatively brief parental education for delayed sleep onset problems in children with ASD was equally effective whether delivered to the parents individually or in groups.

A recent unpublished study by Wiggs and Stores explored the efficacy of behavioural treatment for severe bedtime and night-waking sleep problems in school-age children with ASD. The main issue was whether, given the children's social and communication difficulties, resistance to change, high levels of anxiety and challenging behaviour, this approach would be as effective as it is in normally developing children. Briefly, despite these reservations about the outcome, the parents reported that their children's sleep had improved significantly and that this was still the case 6–8 months later. The children's behaviour at home was also said to have improved. The fact that actigraphically the children's sleep had generally not changed following treatment was interpreted to suggest that a general reduction in tension and friction at home might have altered the parents' general view of the situation.

Regarding pharmacological treatment (Johnson & Malow, 2008), the place of melatonin in the treatment of insomnia, including in children with a neurodevelopmental disorder, was discussed earlier. Doubts have been expressed about the enthusiastic claims for melatonin, mainly because of shortcomings in the scope and design of many studies. In some instances, melatonin has been administered in combination with sleep hygiene advice and behavioural methods, making the reason behind improved sleep difficult to ascertain. However, a number of positive reports concerning children with ASD in particular have been published (Guenole et al., 2011; Rossignol & Frye, 2013) although the reported degree of improvement and the methodological sophistication of the studies have varied.

There is a need for further study of other claims concerning the treatment of sleep disturbance of children with ASD such as the value of clonidine (Ming et al., 2008) and of iron supplements for those ASD children shown to be iron deficient (Dosman et al., 2007). Cortese et al. (2012) concluded that stimulant drugs may be effective for attention deficit hyperactivity disorder-like symptoms in patients with ASD. The place and feasibility of other sleep treatments, such as chronotherapy and light therapy for circadian sleep–wake disorders, in children with ASD is not possible to judge in general terms because of inadequate study. Additional treatments are called for if comorbid conditions, such as epilepsy, are present.

Sleep disturbance in ASD has been accorded high priority in recommendations for paediatric sleep research (Mindell et al., 2006). It is reasonable to expect that, as in the case of other children with a neurodevelopmental disorder, reduction in the sleep disturbance of children with ASD can be followed by improved daytime behaviour (including that of a challenging type) and in mothers' sleep, stress levels and general well-being.

Asperger syndrome

The classification of Asperger syndrome within the autistic spectrum has been debated but, as mentioned earlier, in DSM-5 the condition is now merged within the overall category of ASD.

Studies of sleep problems in Asperger syndrome are few. This is evident from some small-scale earlier reports (Richdale, 2001) as well as more recent accounts. Insomnia has been said to be common in children with Asperger syndrome (Allik et al. 2006; Richdale & Schreck, 2009; Souders et al. 2009), and comparable findings have been reported in adults with this disorder (Hare et al., 2006). A wider range of sleep problems has also been described, such as sleep-related fears, short duration sleep and excessive sleepiness (Paavonen et al., 2008).There is some indication that children diagnosed with Asperger syndrome might have more symptoms of sleep disturbance and different types of sleep problems (including being sluggish and disorientated on waking) than children with a diagnosis of autism who responded better to behavioural treatment (Polimeni et al., 2005). At present, it seems appropriate to follow basically the same assessment and treatment principles that apply with ASD in general.

Allik H, Larsson JO, Smedie H. (2006). Insomnia in school-age children with Asperger syndrome or high-functioning autism. *BMC Psychiatry*, **6**, 18.

Baker E, Richdale A, Short M, Gradisar M. (2013). An investigation of sleep patterns in adolescents with high-functioning autism spectrum disorder compared with typically developing adolescents. *Dev Neurorehabil*, **16**, 155–65.

Charman T, Pickles A, Simonoff E et al. (2011). IQ in children with autism spectrum disorders: data from the Special Needs and Autism Project (SNAP). *Psychol Med*, **41**, 619–27.

Cortese S, Castelnau P, Morcillo C, Roux S, Bonnet-Brilhault F. (2012). Psychostimulants for ADHD-like symptoms in individuals with autism spectrum disorders. *Expert Rev Neurother*, **12**, 461–73.

Cortesi F, Giannotti F, Ivenenko A, Johnson K. (2010). Sleep in children with autistic spectrum disorder. *Sleep Med*, **11**, 659–64.

Cotton S, Richdale A. (2006). Brief report: parental descriptions of sleep problems in children with autism, Down syndrome, and Prader–Willi syndrome. *Res Dev Disabil*, **27**, 151–61.

Dosman CF, Brian JA, Drmic IE *et al*. (2007). Children with autism: effect of iron supplementation on sleep and ferritin. *Pediatr Neurol*, **36**, 152–8.

Giannotti F, Cortesi F, Cerquiglini, A, Vagnoni C, Valente D. (2011). Sleep in children with autism with and without autistic regression. *J Sleep Res*, **20**, 338–47.

Glickman G. (2009). Circadian rhythms and sleep in children with autism. *Neurosci Biobehav Rev*, **34**, 755–68.

Goldman SE, Richdale AL, Clemons T, Malow BA. (2011). Parental sleep concerns in autism spectrum disorders: variations from childhood to adolescence. *J Autism Dev Disord*, **42**, 531–8.

Goodlin-Jones BL, Tang K, Liu J, Anders TF. (2008). Sleep patterns in preschool-age children with autism, developmental delay, and typical development. *J Am Acad Child Adolesc Psychiatry*, **47**, 930–8.

Guenole F, Godbout R, Nicolas A *et al*. (2011). Melatonin for disordered sleep in individuals with autism spectrum disorders: systematic review and discussion. *Sleep Med Rev*, **15**, 379–87.

Hare DJ, Jones S, Evershed K. (2006). A comparative study of circadian rhythm functioning and sleep in people with Asperger syndrome. *Autism*, **10**, 565–75.

Hollway JA, Aman MG. (2011). Sleep correlates of pervasive developmental disorders: a review of the literature. *Rev Dev Disabil*, **32**, 1399–421.

Humphreys JS, Gringras P, Blair PS *et al*. (2014). Sleep patterns in children with autistic spectrum disorders: a prospective cohort study. *Arch Dis Child*, **99**, 114–18.

Jeste SS. (2011). The neurology of autism spectrum disorders. *Curr Opin Neurol*, **24**, 132–9.

Johnson CR, Turner KS, Foldes E *et al*. (2013). Behavioral parent training to address sleep disturbances in young children with autism spectrum disorder: a pilot trial. *Sleep Med*, **14**, 995–1004.

Johnson KP, Giannotti F, Cortesi F. (2009). Sleep patterns in autism spectrum disorders. *Child Adolesc Psychiatr Clin N Am*, **18**, 917–28.

Johnson KP, Malow BA. (2008). Assessment and pharmacologic treatment of sleep disturbance in autism. *Child Adolesc Psychiatr Clin N Am*, **17**, 773–85.

Joshi G, Petty C, Wosniak J *et al*. (2010). The heavy burden of psychiatric comorbidity in youth with autism spectrum disorders: a large comparative study of a psychiatrically referred population. *J Autism Dev Disord*, **40**, 1361–70.

Krakowiak P, Goodlin-Jones B, Hertz-Picciotto I, Croen LA, Hansen RL. (2008). Sleep problems in children with autism spectrum disorders, developmental delays, and typical development: a population-based study. *J Sleep Res*, **17**, 197–206.

Kulman G, Lissoni P, Rovelli F. (2000). Evidence of pineal hypofunction in autistic children. *Neuro Endocrinol Lett*, **21**, 31–4.

Leyfer OT, Folstein SE, Bacalman S *et al*. (2006). Comorbid psychiatric disorders in children with autism: interview development and rates of disorders. *J Autism Dev Disord*, **36**, 849–61.

Lopez-Wagner MC, Hoffman CD, Sweeney DP, Hodge D, Gilliam JE. (2008). Sleep problems of parents of typically developing children and parents of children with autism. *Genet Psychol*, **169**, 245–59.

Malow BA. (2004). Sleep disorders, epilepsy, and autism. *Ment Retard Dev Disabil Res Rev*, **10**, 122–5.

Malow BA, Adkins KW, Reynolds A *et al.* (2014). Parent –based sleep education for children with autism spectrum disorders. *J Autism Dev Disord*, **44**, 216–28.

Malow BA, Byars K, Johnson K. (2012). A practice pathway for the identification, evaluation, and management of insomnia in children and adolescents with autistic spectrum disorders. *Pediatrics*, **130** Suppl 2, S106–24.

Malow BA, Marsec ML, McGrew SG. (2006). Characterising sleep in children with autism spectrum disorders: a multidimensional approach. *Sleep*, **29**, 1563–71.

Maski KP, Jeste SS, Spence SJ. (2011). Common neurological co-morbidities in autism spectrum disorders. *Curr Opin Pediatr*, **23**, 609–15.

Matson JL, Rieske RD, Williams LW. (2013). The relationship between autism spectrum disorders and attention/hyperactivity disorder: an overview. *Res Dev Disabil*, **34**, 2475–84.

Meltzer LJ (2008). Brief report; sleep in parents of children with autism spectrum disorders. *Pediatr Psychol*, **33**, 380–6.

Miano S, Bruni O, Elia M *et al.* (2007). Sleep in children with autistic spectrum disorder: a questionnaire and polysomnographic study. *Sleep Med*, **9**, 64–70.

Miano S, Ferri R. (2010). Epidemiology and management of insomnia in children with autistic spectrum disorders. *Paediatr Drugs*, **12**, 75–84.

Mindell JA, Emslie G, Blumer J *et al.* (2006). Pharmacological management of insomnia in children and adolescents: consensus statement. *Pediatrics*, **117**, e1223–32.

Ming X, Gordon E, Kang N, Wagner GC. (2008). Use of clonidine in children with autism spectrum disorders. *Brain Dev*, **30**, 454–60.

Ming X, Sun Y-M, Nachajon RV, Brimacombe M, Walters AS. (2009). Prevalence of parasomnia in autistic children with sleep disorders. *Clin Med Pediatr*, **3**, 1–10.

Murray ML, Hsia Y, Glaser K *et al.* (2013). Pharmacological treatments prescribed to people with autism spectrum disorder (ASD) in primary health care. *Psychopharmacology (Berl)*, May 17 PMID: 23681164

Paavonen EJ, Vehkalahti K, Vanhala R *et al.* (2008). Sleep in children with Asperger syndrome. *J Autism Dev Disord*, **38**, 41–51.

Parrino L, Ferri R, Bruni O, Terzano MG. (2012). Cyclic alternating pattern (CAP): the marker of sleep instability. *Sleep Med Rev*, **16**, 27–45.

Polimeni MA, Richdale AL, Francis AJ. (2005). A survey of sleep problems in autism, Asperger's disorder and typically developing children. *J Intellect Disabil Res*, **49** (Pt 4), 260–8.

Reynolds AM, Malow BA. (2011). Sleep and autism spectrum disorders. *Pediatr Clin North Am*, **58**, 685–98.

Richdale A. Sleep in children with autism and Asperger syndrome. In: Stores G, Wiggs L, eds. *Sleep disturbance in Children and Adolescents with Disorders of Development: Its Significance and Management*. London: Mac Keith Press 2001. 181–91.

Richdale AL, Schreck KA. (2009). Sleep problems in autism spectrum disorders: prevalence, nature & possible biopsychosocial aetiologies. *Sleep Med Rev*, **13**, 403–11.

Rossignol DA, Frye RE. (2013). Melatonin in autism spectrum disorders. *Curr Clin Pharmacol*,[Epub ahead of print]

Santangelo SL, Tsatsanis K. (2005). What is known about autism,: genes, brain, and behavior. *Am J Pharmacogenomics*, **5**, 71–92.

Schreck KA, Mulick JA. (2000). Parental report of sleep problems in children with autism. *J Autis Dev Disord*, **30**, 127–35.

Sikora DM, Johnson K, Clemons T, Katz T. (2012). The relationship between sleep problems and daytime behavior in children of different ages with autism spectrum disorders. *Pediatrics*, **130** Suppl 2, S83–90.

Silver WG, Rapin I. (2012). Neurological basis of autism. *Pediatr Clin North Am*, **59**, 45–61.

Simonoff E, Jones CR, Baird G *et al.* (2013). The persistence and stability of psychiatric problems in adolescents with autism spectrum disorders. *J Child Psychol Psychiatry*, **54**, 186–94.

Simonoff E, Jones CR, Pickles A *et al.* (2012). Severe mood problems in adolescents with autism spectrum disorder. *J Child Psychol Psychiatry*, **53**, 1157–66.

Simonoff E, Pickles A, Charman T *et al.* (2008). Psychiatric disorders in children with autism spectrum disorders: prevalence, comorbidity, and associated factors in a population-derived sample. *J Am Acad Child Adolesc Psychiatry*, **47**, 921–9.

Skokauskas N, Gallagher L. (2012). Mental Health aspects of autistic spectrum disorders in children. *J Intellect Disabil Res*, **56**, 248–57.

Souders MC, Mason TB, Valladares O *et al.* (2009). Sleep behaviours and sleep quality in children with autism spectrum disorders. *Sleep*, **32**, 1566–78.

Thirumalai SS, Shubin RA, Robinson R. (2002). Rapid eye movement sleep behavior disorder in children with autism. *J Child Neurol*, **17**, 173–8.

Vriend JL, Corkum PV, Moon EC, Smith IM. (2011). Behavioral interventions for sleep problems in children with autism spectrum disorders: current findings and future directions. *J Pediatr Psychol*, **36**, 1017–29.

Wengel T, Hanlon-Dearman AC, Fjeldsted B. (2011). Sleep and sensory characteristics in young children with fetal alcohol spectrum disorder. *J Dev Behav Pediatr*, **32**, 384–92.

Wiggs L, Stores G. (2004). Sleep patterns and sleep disorders in children with Autistic spectrum disorders: insights using parent report and actigraphy. *Dev Med Child Neurol*, **46**, 372–80.

Youssef J, Singh K, Huntington N, Becker R, Kothare SV. (2013). Relationship of serum ferritin levels to sleep fragmentation and periodic limb movements of sleep on polysomnography in autism spectrum disorders. *Pediatr Neurol*, **49**, 274–8.

Zafeiriou DI, Ververi A, Vargiami E. (2007). Childhood autism and associated comorbidities. *Brain Dev*, **29**, 257–72.

Attention deficit hyperactivity disorder (ADHD)

'ADHD' is a long-standing but still troublesome concept. Dr Heinrich Hoffman gave a vivid account of ADHD-type behaviour in his 1845 *The Story of Fidgety Philip* (Hoffman, 2000) (see Box 8). However, Barkley and Peters (2012) argue that the first description of 'attention deficit' was by Weikard, a German physician, in 1775. In more recent times, various medical terms have been used such as 'minimal brain dysfunction' and 'hyperkinetic reaction of childhood', although some still contend that it is not a medical condition at all, that instead it is merely a 'social construct'. Counter to this belief are reports of genetic and neuroimaging abnormalities associated with some children with ADHD. As there is no diagnostic test, recognition relies on subjective reports about behaviour. ADHD is included in the DSM-5 section on neurodevelopmental disorders. As indicated in various parts of this chapter, ADHD is commonly described as an accompaniment of many different neurodevelopmental disorders.

Three basic subtypes have been described: predominantly inattentive, predominantly hyperkinetic-impulsive, and combined. The severe form of the combined subtype corresponds to the ICD-10 condition called 'hyperkinetic disorder'. The subtype exhibited by any one person may vary over time. Defined in DSM terms, ADHD is said to occur in 3–5% of school-age children and adolescents, mainly males. By comparison, the prevalence of ICD 'hyperkinetic disorder' is given as 1–2%.

Comprehensive reviews of the published work on sleep and ADHD to which the reader is referred for detailed information include those by Owens (2009); Gruber (2009); Spruyt and Gozal (2011); and Yoon *et al.* (2012). The following account aims to simply highlight aspects of basic clinical importance. The intricacies and uncertainties concerning the relationships between ADHD and sleep are reflected in the various suggestions for further research discussed by Owens *et al.* (2013).

Box 8 ADHD

The Story of Fidgety Philip is from a book of children's poems called *Struwwelpeter* written and illustrated by Heinrich Hoffman, a German psychiatrist, in 1844. The poems were intended to teach children about the serious consequences of misbehaviour.

Fidgety Philip's behaviour is thought to be one of the earliest accounts of attention deficit hyperactivity disorder. The following is an extract from the poem.

> See the naughty, restless child,
> Growing still more rude and wild,
> Till his chair falls over quite.
> Philip screams with all his might,
> Catches at the cloth, but then
> That makes matters worse again.
> Down upon the ground they fall,
> Glasses, bread, knives, forks and all.
> How Mamma did fret and frown,
> When she saw them tumbling down!
> And Papa made such a face!
> Philip is in sad disgrace.

Hoffman H. *Struwwelpeter in English Translation*. Dover Children's Books. New York: Dover Publications 2000.

Occurrence of sleep disturbance in ADHD
The reviews just mentioned all point out the complexities and unresolved issues concerning the subject of sleep and ADHD, not least of which concerns the problem that there is a reciprocal relationship between the two in that sleep loss or poor quality sleep can give rise to ADHD-type symptoms while ADHD can disturb sleep (see later). There is, however, agreement that parents commonly report that their children diagnosed as having ADHD have sleep problems well in excess of children in general, estimates ranging up to 50% or more.

Types of sleep disturbance
Parental reports of sleep problems usually take the usual forms of insomnia, i.e. bedtime struggles because of the child's refusal to settle to sleep, delay in getting to sleep, troublesome night wakings, restless sleep and early morning awakening without returning to sleep. In addition to insomnia, many other types of sleep disturbance have been reported (Walters *et al.*, 2008; Konofal *et al.* 2010). These include restless sleep, excessive daytime sleepiness, restless legs syndrome, periodic limb movements in sleep, rhythmic movement disorder such as headbanging, sleep apnoea, parasomnias such as arousal disorders, sleep apnoea, narcolepsy, and circadian rhythm disorders such as delayed sleep–wake phase disorder. Chiang *et al.* (2010) described different patterns of sleep disturbance in the three ADHD subtypes mentioned above. In their series the combined and predominantly hyperkinetic-impulsive subtypes were associated with circadian sleep–wake problems, sleep talking and nightmares; the predominantly inattentive subtype was associated with hypersomnia.

Factors potentially contributing to sleep disturbance
An appreciation of the many possible ways in which the sleep of children with ADHD can become disturbed is essential for appropriate investigation and management of their sleep problems. The following may at least be contributory factors.

Pathophysiological. Central nervous system processes (especially involving the prefrontal cortex) are common to sleep and also the regulation of attention and arousal. It has been suggested that there may be a subgroup of children with ADHD with a circadian sleep phase delay and delayed onset of melatonin secretion, and that ADHD is associated with a hypo-arousal state (Golan *et al.*, 2004) which the affected child's increased activity levels serves to counteract. The evidence of genetic influences in ADHD also points to the relevance of intrinsic factors (Khan & Faraone, 2006). Of the range of children diagnosed with ADHD, intellectual impairment can be a feature, especially in those with the type corresponding to ICD 'hyperkinetic disorder' where comorbid medical disorders affecting the brain (including epilepsy and certain neurodevelopmental disorders) are present (Taylor, 2006).

Physical comorbidities. Epilepsy may be associated with ADHD in the various ways discussed by Hamoda *et al.* (2009) although the underlying mechanisms are ill-defined. An association between low serum ferritin levels and sleep disturbance on children with ADHD has been suggested (eg. Abou-Khadra *et al.*, 2013) but this supposed link has been debated (Donfrancesco *et al.*, 2013).

Psychiatric comorbidities. About 70% of children described as having ADHD have a comorbid psychiatric disorder (Mayes *et al.* 2009) such as oppositional defiant or conduct disorder, anxiety disorder, and depression, all of which are potentially associated with disturbed sleep. Such associations were said to be least in the inattentive type of ADHD. Autistic symptoms have also been described as common in association with ADHD (Reiersen & Todd, 2008). Matson *et al.* (2013) have considered the complexities of the relationship between ADHD and ASD.

Medication effects. Possibilities include the effects of stimulant drugs which in some children with ADHD cause insomnia, restless sleep or disturbance of circadian rhythms (Ironside *et al.* 2010), and 'rebound hyperactivity' at bedtime can occur as the effects of daytime delivered stimulant medication wears off. Other possible medication effects on sleep are discussed in Chapter 1.

Parenting. Sleep disturbance can pose considerable problems for the child, parents and the family in general (Sung *et al.*, 2008) and parents may well find it a greater challenge than coping with their child's disruptive behaviour during the day. Good sleep hygiene principles or behavioural methods of treating insomnia may well be particularly difficult for parents to implement because of their emotional state. The acquisition of good sleep habits can be hampered not only by inappropriate parenting practices but also the child's behavioural problems or learning difficulties. In general, few objective sleep abnormalities have been demonstrated compared with the frequency of parents' complaints about their child's sleep (Wiggs *et al.*, 2005). Conceivably, this is explained by parents' tendency to overstate the extent of the problems because of their heightened emotional condition.

Associated neurodevelopmental disorders. Hyperkinetic disorder in particular can also be associated with other neurodevelopmental disorders such as ASD and a number of other conditions discussed in this chapter.

Sleep assessment

Hysing (2014) has made recommendations to guide the assessment and the management of sleep disorders in ADHD. Reference has already been made to the reciprocal relationship between sleep and ADHD. In the various ways just suggested, ADHD may cause sleep disturbance. Alternatively, ADHD behaviours can be the result of primary sleep disorders. Any sleep disorder causing inadequate or disrupted, poor quality sleep can produce ADHD-type symptoms because, unlike adults in whom such sleep disturbance usually causes a reduction of activity levels, children can react in the opposite way. Ideally it is important to determine whether or not a sleep disorder preceded the onset of ADHD symptoms. Coexisting sleep disturbance may worsen ADHD symptoms already present for other reasons. The particular sleep disorders implicated in these ways have included sleep apnoea, restless legs syndrome, periodic limb movement disorder, circadian sleep–wake cycle disorders and narcolepsy (Chervin *et al.*, 2002; Walters *et al.*, 2008; Youssef *et al.*, 2011). Treatment of these conditions has been reported to lead to a reduction of ADHD symptoms.

As such a variety of factors (acting singly or in combination) can be responsible for the development of ADHD-type behaviour, a comprehensive approach is needed in an attempt to identify the reasons for sleep disturbance in children said to have this condition. First, however, in view of the varied use of the term ADHD, there is merit in assessing the behaviour of such children in order to confirm the diagnosis and identify its subtype. This can be done by using the DSM-IV ADHD Rating Scale completed by parents and teachers (DuPaul *et al.*, 1998).

Screening for sleep disturbance
Because any sleep disorder causing inadequate or disrupted sleep can paradoxically produce ADHD-type behaviours in children, all children for whom the diagnosis of ADHD has been considered (whether by strict diagnostic criteria or otherwise) should be screened for possible sleep disturbance, especially sleep disordered breathing (Youssef *et al.*, 2011). As in other neurodevelopmental disorders, it is appropriate to do this not only initially but also at intervals during each child's care in case the situation has changed since the last assessment. The means of achieving this is described in Chapter 1.

Diagnosis
When screening suggests a sleep problem, the exact nature of the underlying disorder(s) and contributory factors needs to be identified (see Chapter 1). In outline, ADHD-type behaviour can be considered to be: ADHD (a) as formally diagnosed by DSM criteria; (b) as a result of a primary sleep disorder; (c) as a consequence of sleep disturbance caused by comorbid medical or behavioural/psychiatric disorder, or other neurodevelopmental disorder; or (d) attributable to medication. Owens (2009) provides an algorithm for comprehensively assessing such possible causes or contributory factors.

Aspects of management
As mentioned earlier, Hysing (2014) has suggested guidelines for both the assessment and management of sleep disorders in ADHD. Corkum *et al.* (2011) emphasize that choice of treatment depends on the results of assessing the nature and cause of the sleep disturbance in children with ADHD. Improvement in sleep by whatever means may well help to reduce ADHD symptoms. The standard behavioural treatments for sleep disturbance in children in general (described in Chapter 1) can be employed. Promotion of good sleep hygiene alone may reduce bedtime sleep problems in children with ADHD (Owens, 2009) but in any case it should be combined with whatever other form of treatment is used.

In their review, Barrett *et al.* (2013) point to the shortage of evidence concerning pharmacological treatment specifically for ADHD related sleep disorders. They suggest that clonidine and melatonin have something in their favour for insomnia problems but behavioural methods are recommended by Hoebert *et al.* (2009), possibly combined with melatonin in severe cases or where the sleep problem appears to be intrinsic. Weiss *et al.* (2006) reported the combination of sleep hygiene and melatonin to be effective for difficulty settling to sleep in children with ADHD taking stimulant medication.

Konofal *et al.* (2010) include the contributions of comorbidities in their discussion of the management of possible sleep disorders underlying the ADHD. Guidance on the treatment of epilepsy in children has been provided by Aldenkamp *et al* (2006). Pliszka (2003) has considered the management implications of psychiatric comorbidities in particular. Reiersen and Todd (2008) suggested that the coexistence of ASD with ADHD might limit the value of standard ADHD treatment, but Cortese *et al.* (2012) were rather more optimistic than this.

Regular follow-up for review is essential as clinical circumstances may well change in the course of the child's development. As an example, Landberg *et al.* (2014), having found associations between self-reported daytime sleepiness in college students with ADHD and impaired aspects of their academic and overall functioning, stress the importance of monitoring and treating their sleep disturbances. As childhood ADHD often persists at least partially into adulthood (Rosler *et al.*, 2010), long-term follow-up arrangements need to be considered.

Abou-Khadra MK, Amin OR, Shaker OG, Rabah TM. (2013). Parent-reported sleep problems, symptom ratings, and serum ferritin levels in children with attention-deficit/hyperactivity disorder: a case control study. *BMC Pediatr*, **13**, 217.

Aldenkamp AP, Arzimanoglou A, Reijs R, Van Mil S. (2006). Optimising therapy of seizures in children and adolescents with ADHD. *Neurology*, **67** (Suppl 4), S49–51.

Barkley RA, Peters H. (2012). The earliest reference to ADHD in the medical literature? Melchior Adam Weikard's description in 1775 of "attention deficit" (Mangel der Aufmerksamkeit, Attentio Volubilis). *J Atten Disord*, **16**, 623–30.

Barrett JR, Tracy DK, Giaroli G. (2013). To sleep or not to sleep: a systematic review of the literature of pharmacological treatments of insomnia in children and adolescents with attention-deficit/hyperactivity disorder. *J Child Adolesc Psychopharmacol*, **23**, 640–7.

Chervin RD, Archbold KH, Dillon JE *et al.* (2002). Associations between symptoms of inattention, hyperactivity, restless legs, and periodic leg movements. *Sleep*, **25**, 213–18.

Chiang HL, Gau SS, Ni HC *et al.* (2010). Association between symptoms and subtypes of attention-deficit hyperactivity disorder and sleep problems/disorders. *J Sleep Res*, **19**, 535–45.

Corkum P, Davidson F, Macpherson M. (2011). A framework for assessment and treatment of sleep problems in children with attention-deficit/ hyperactivity disorder. *Pediatr Clin North Am*, **58**, 667–83.

Cortese S, Castelnau P, Morcillo C, Roux S, Bonnet-Brilhault F. (2012). Psychostimulants for ADHD-like symptoms in individuals with autism spectrum disorders. *Expert Rev. Neurother*, **12**, 461–73.

Donfrancesco R, Parisi P, Vanacore N *et al.* (2013). Iron and ADHD: time to move beyond serum ferritin levels. *J Atten Disord*, **17**, 347–57.

DuPaul GJ, Power T, Anastopoulos AD, Reid R. *ADHD Rating Scale*. New York: Guilford Press 1998.

Golan N, Shahar E, Ravid S, Pillar G. (2004). Sleep disorders and daytime sleepiness in children with attention-deficit/hyperactive disorder. *Sleep*, **27**, 261–6.

Gruber R. (2009). Sleep characteristics of children and adolescents with attention deficit-hyperactivity disorder. *Child Adolesc Psychiatr Clin N Am*, **18**, 863–76.

Hamoda HM, Guild DJ, Gumlak S, Travers BH, Gonzalez-Heydrich J. (2009). Association between attention-deficit/hyperactivity disorder and epilepsy in pediatric populations. *Expert Rev Neurother*, **9**, 1747–54.

Hoebert M, van der Heijden KB, van Geijlswijk IM, Smits MG. (2009). Long-term follow up of melatonin treatment in children with ADHD and chronic sleep onset insomnia. *J Pineal Res*, **47**, 1–7.

Hysing M. (2014). Review: recommendations for the assessment and management of sleep disorders in ADHD. *Evid Based Ment Health*, **17**,

Ironside S, Davidson F, Corkum P. (2010). Circadian motor activity affected by stimulant medication in children with attention-deficit/hyperactivity disorder. *J Sleep Res*, **19**, 546–51.

Khan SA, Faraone SV. (2006). The genetics of ADHD: a literature review of 2005. *Curr Psychiatry Rep*, **8**, 393–7.

Konofal E, Lecendreux M, Cortese S. (2010). Sleep and ADHD. *Sleep Med*, **11**, 652–8.

Landberg JM, Dvorsky MR, Becker SP, Mollitor SJ. (2014). The impact of daytime sleepiness on the school performance of college students with attention deficit hyperactivity disorder (ADHD): a prospective longitudinal study. *J Sleep Res*, **23**, 318–25.

Matson JL, Rieske RD, Williams LW. (2013). The relationship between autism spectrum disorders and attention/hyperactivity disorder: an overview. *Res Dev Disabil*, **34**, 2475–84.

Mayes SD, Calhoun SL, Bixler EO *et al.* (2009). ADHD subtypes and comorbid anxiety, depression, and oppositional-defiant disorder: differences in sleep problems. *J Pediatr Psychol*, **34**, 328–37.

Owens J, Gruber R, Brown T *et al.* (2013). Future research directions in sleep and ADHD: report of a consensus working group. *J Atten Disord*, **17**, 550–64.

Owens JA. (2009). A clinical overview of sleep and attention-deficit/hyperactivity disorder in children and adolescents. *J Can Acad Child Adolesc Psychiatry*, **18**, 92–102.

Pliszka SR. (2003). Psychiatric comorbidities in children with attention deficit hyperactivity disorder: implications for management. *Pediatr Drugs*, **5**, 741–50.

Reiersen AM, Todd RD. (2008). Co-occurrence of ADHD and autism spectrum disorders: phenomenology and treatment. *Expert Rev Neurother*, **8**, 657–69.

Rosler M, Casas M, Konofal E, Buitelaar J. (2010). Attention deficit hyperactivity disorder in adults. *World J Biol Psychiatry*, **11**, 684–98.

Spruyt K, Gozal D. (2011). Sleep disturbances in children with attention-deficit/hyperactivity disorder. *Expert Rev Neurother*, **11**, 565–77.

Sung V, Hiscock H, Sciberras E, Efron D. (2008). Sleep problems in children with attention-deficit/hyperactivity disorder: prevalence and the effect on the family. *Arch Pediatr Adolesc Med*, **162**, 336–42.

Taylor E. Hyperkinetic disorders. In: Gillberg C, Harrington R, Steinhausen H-C, eds. *A Clinician's Handbook of Child and Adolescent Psychiatry*. Cambridge: Cambridge University Press 2006, 489–521.

Walters AS, Silvestri R, Zucconi M, Chandrashekaria R, Konofal E. (2008). Review of the possible relationship and hypothetical links between attention deficit hyperactivity disorder (ADHD) and the simple sleep related movement disorders, parasomnias, hypersomnias, and circadian rhythm disorders. *J Clin Sleep Med*, **4**, 591–600.

Weiss MD, Wasdell MB, Bomben MM, Rea KJ, Freeman RD. (2006). Sleep hygiene and melatonin treatment for children and adolescents with ADHD and initial insomnia. *J Am Acad Child Adolesc Psychiatry*, **45**, 512–19.

Wiggs L, Montgomery P, Stores G. (2005). Actigraphic and parent reports of sleep patterns and sleep disorders in children with subtypes of attention-deficit hyperactivity disorder. *Sleep*, **28**, 1437–45.

Yoon SYR, Jain U, Shapiro C. (2012). Sleep in attention-deficit/hyperactivity disorder in children and adults: Past, present, and future. *Sleep Med Rev*, **16**, 371–88.

Youssef NA, Ege M, Angly SS, Strauss JL, Marx CE. (2011). Is obstructive sleep apnea associated with ADHD? *Ann Clin Psychiatry*, **23**, 213–24.

Tourette syndrome (TS)

This disorder is characterized by multiple motor tics and one or more vocal tics. Genetic and environmental factors are considered to play a part in the condition but its exact causes are not known. The modern view of TS has been comprehensively reviewed by Robertson (2012) who gives the worldwide prevalence as 1% with a few geographical exceptions.

Sleep disturbance

The above review mentions that that tics can occur in sleep and that sleep disturbance is a common difficulty. Sleep aspects of TS have been more generally discussed elsewhere, especially by Rothenberger *et al.* (2001). Consistently since the 1980s and up to the present day, disturbed sleep patterns have been described in children with TS. This appears to be particularly so in the large majority of cases with both TS and attention deficit hyperactivity disorder (Kirov *et al.*, 2007). Severity of the condition is also important: marked tics can interfere with getting to sleep and staying asleep; lesser tics during sleep may not be so disruptive.

Types of sleep disturbance

A wide range of sleep disturbances has been described (Rothenburger *et al.*, 2001): difficulties falling asleep, frequent awakenings at night, restless sleep, a number of parasomnias (e.g. sleepwalking, sleep talking, nightmares) and sleep apnoea, as well as restless legs syndrome and also periodic limb movements during sleep. REM sleep behaviour disorder has also been described in a child with TS (Trajanovic *et al.*, 2004). A number of these problems and disorders predispose to excessive daytime sleepiness because of reduction or impairment of overnight sleep and, indeed, polysomnographic studies have shown some evidence of reduced sleep efficiency (percentage of time in bed spent asleep), as well as reduction of deep NREM and REM sleep.

Factors potentially contributing to sleep disturbance

Pathophysiological. Based on their polysomnographic findings and other intensive monitoring of young people with TS, an intrinsic disorder of arousal was suggested by Kostanecka-Endress *et al.* (2003) who considered that this increased arousal phenomenon might trigger tics and other behavioural problems during the day. However, its nature seems to have remained ill-defined. The same is true for other possible structural and neurophysiological including neurotransmitter systems (Singer, 2005) further details of which are reviewed by Robertson (2012). Cortese *et al.* (2008) suggested that iron deficiency, by its action on catecholamine metabolism, might explain comorbidity of TS, attention deficit hyperactivity disorder and restless legs syndrome. Intellectual levels are generally normal in TS.

Physical comorbidities. It has been suggested that that headaches are commonly present in children with TS, especially migraine headaches and tension-type headaches (Ghosh *et al.*, 2012), but this has not been generally accepted as established.

Psychiatric comorbidities. Accounts of comorbidities in TS have very largely been concerned with comorbid psychiatric conditions. Robertson (2012) quotes an international survey of 3500 patients of all ages with TS which indicated that 88% were reported to have comorbidities many of which are capable of disturbing sleep in their different ways. Attention deficit hyperactivity disorder, obsessive-compulsive disorder and autism spectrum disorder predominate. Robertson suggests that much of the genetic susceptibility for TS may be shared with these other disorders, constituting a general genetic susceptibility which is then influenced by specific genes and environmental factors to produce one or other of these neuro-developmental disorders.

Other coexisting psychopathological conditions associated with TS and capable disturbing sleep include depression, anxiety, oppositional defiant disorder, conduct disorder and personality disorder. Throughout, the combination of TS and attention deficit hyperactivity disorder is seen to particularly predispose to such psychiatric problems and their consequences, presumably including effects on sleep. Frequent arousals from sleep are reported to be associated with problem behaviours in children with TS, whether or not associated with attention deficit hyperactivity disorder (Stephens *et al.* 2013). The presence of obsessive-compulsive disorder is associated with social and educational difficulties, as well as impaired quality of life in children with TS (Bernard *et al.*, 2009; Debes *et al.*, 2010), potentially adding to emotional problems.

Medication effects. Robertson's 2012 review of current medications used for TS (mainly antipsychotics) includes drugs which might, for example, cause daytime sleepiness.

Parenting. Reports by Cooper *et al.* (2003) and Lee *et al.* (2007) demonstrate that TS, including its comorbidities, causes parents considerable stress and mental health problems. Robertson (2012) enlarges on this point in her review of a number of studies which have demonstrated the effects of TS on caregiver burden and parenting stress as well as affected children's quality of life. In these circumstances, parenting ability, including encouraging their children to acquire good sleep habits, is highly likely to be impaired.

Aspects of assessment and management

As in other neurodevelopmental disorders (perhaps more than most) a comprehensive, multidisciplinary approach to diagnosis and treatment in TS is required, guided by the general principles described earlier. However, in view of the common comorbidity of TS and attention deficit hyperactivity disorder, and the psychiatric and psychosocial complications (to which can be added the implications for sleep) of the latter, attention has been paid increasingly to pharmacological treatment of this combination. Rizzo *et al.* (2013) provisionally concluded from their revue that clonidine might be the first line of treatment with atomoxetine or methylphenidate as alternatives.

Bernard BA, Stebbins GT, Siegel S *et al.* (2009). Determinants of quality of life in children with Gilles de la Tourette syndrome. *Mov Disord*, **24**, 1070–3.

Cooper C, Robertson MM, Livingstone G. (2003). Psychological morbidity and caregiver burden in parents of children with Tourette's disorder and psychiatric comorbidity. *J Am Acad Child Adolesc Psychiatry*, **42**, 1370–5.

Cortese S, Lescendreaux M, Bernadina BD *et al.* (2008). Attention-deficit/hyperactivity disorder, Tourette's syndrome, and restless legs syndrome: the iron hypothesis. *Med Hypotheses*, **70**, 1128–32.

Debes N, Hjalgrim H, Skov L. (2010). The presence of attention-deficit hyperactivity disorder (ADHD) and obsessive-compulsive disorder worsen psychosocial and educational problems in Tourette syndrome. *J Child Neurol*, **25**, 171–81.

Ghosh D, Rajan PV, Das D *et al.* (2012). Headache in children with Tourette syndrome. *J Pediatr*, **161**, 303–7.

Kirov R, Kinkelbur J, Banaschewski T, Rothenberger A. (2007). Sleep patterns in children with attention-deficit/hyperactivity disorder, tic disorder, and comorbidity. *J Child Psychol Psychiatry*, **48**, 561–70.

Kostanecka-Endress T, Banaschewski T, Kinkelbur J. (2003). Disturbed sleep in children with Tourette syndrome: a polysomnographic study. *J Psychosomatic Res*, **55**, 23–9.

Lee MY, Chen YC, Wang HS, Chen DR. (2007). Parenting stress and related factors in parents of children with Tourette syndrome. *J Nurs Res*, **15**, 165–74.

Rizzo, R, Gulisano M, Cali PV, Curatolo P. (2013). Tourette syndrome and comorbid ADHD: Current pharmacological treatment options. *Eur J Paediatr Neurol*, **17**, 421–8.

Robertson MM. (2012). The Gilles de la Tourette syndrome: the current status. *Arch Dis Educ Pract Ed*, **97**, 166–75.

Rothenberger T, Kostanecka T, Kinkelbur J *et al.* Sleep and Tourette syndrome. In: Cohen DJ, Goetz G, Jancovic J, eds. *Tourette Syndrome*. Philadelphia: Williams and Wilkins 2001. 245–59.

Singer HS. (2005). Tourette's syndrome: from behaviour to biology. *Lancet Neurol*, **4**, 149–59.

Stephens RJ, Chung SA, Jovanovic D *et al.* (2013). Relationship between polysomnographic sleep architecture and behaviour in medication-free children with TS, ADHD, TS and ADHD, and controls. *J Dev Behav Pediatr*, **34**, 688–96.

Trajanovic NN, Voloh I, Shapiro CM, Sandor P. (2004). REM sleep behavior disorder in a child with Tourette's syndrome. *Can J Neurol Sci*, **31**, 572–5.

Chronic fatigue syndrome (CFS)

The review of CFS in children and adolescents by Garralda and Rangel (2002) demonstrated the many uncertainties regarding the nature of the condition (including whether it can be regarded as a medical problem or not), its associations, response to treatment, and its outcome. Biological, genetic, infectious and psychological mechanisms have been proposed but the aetiology of CFS is still not understood and it may have multiple causes. Despite its various alternative names including myalgic encephalomyelitis (ME), it might be questioned whether CFS qualifies as a neuropsychiatric disorder. It is included here because it is generally managed within psychiatric services, its possible neuropathological components and its association with disturbed sleep.

The main features of CFS described by Garralda and Rangel (2002) are severe physical fatigue or exhaustion often accompanied by headaches or muscle pain or discomfort, as well as sleep problems (fatigue or lack of energy is different from excessive sleepiness in that it does not involve the need to sleep). Inactivity may be marked with prolonged bed rest, absence from school and social isolation. Onset is often thought to follow an acute infection or flu-type illness. This disabling condition is said to affect about 0.2% of the population as a whole.

Diagnosis of CFS can present problems. The report by Mariman et al. (2013) that comprehensive, multidisciplinary assessment of a group of adults referred for chronic unexplained fatigue revealed that only a minority met official criteria for the diagnosis of CFS. Of children and adolescents attending a chronic fatigue clinic, 60% (about two-thirds female) were eventually diagnosed as having CFS, often after a long delay. The rest received a psychiatric and/or medical diagnosis. In addition to fatigue, the variety of complaints were sleep disturbance (86%), malaise following physical exertion, pain, and autonomic and cognitive symptoms (Knight et al., 2013).

Sleep disturbance in CFS

Since the early 1990s, disturbed sleep has been reported to be a common part of CFS syndrome with high rates of complaints mainly in the form of insomnia, unrefreshing sleep and daytime sleepiness (Stores, 1999). Relatively few reports have concerned young patients. Ohinata et al. (2008) described evidence in children with CFS of higher rates of abnormal sleep–wake rhythms and disrupted sleep compared with healthy controls, and PSG assessment of teenagers (without other psychiatric disorder) with a formal diagnosis of CFS showed significantly higher levels of both brief and longer awakenings compared with controls (Stores et al., 1998). This poorly sustained sleep (likely to affect its restorative value) was in keeping with the findings in some of adults with CFS, such as that by Sharpley et al. (1997).

In a minority of adults with CFS, detailed enquiry has revealed specific sleep disorders to account for their symptoms, namely sleep apnoea, periodic limb movements in sleep (sometimes with accompanying restless legs syndrome) or narcolepsy (see Stores, 1999). The relationship between fibromyalgia and CFS remains unclear. Recent publications about sleep and mainly adult CFS (Togo *et al.*, 2008; Jackson & Bruck, 2010; Mariman *et al.*, 2013) echo some of the points made in earlier accounts with the addition of more up to date impressions.

Despite the view that CSF is associated with abnormalities of the central and autonomic nervous systems (Komaroff & Cho, 2011), intrinsic neurobiological influences have still not been identified despite sophisticated forms of analysis of sleep physiology, for example. Assessment needs to be based on awareness of various factors associated with childhood CFS which can predispose to sleep disturbance or act as perpetuating influences. These include comorbid psychiatric disorders (mainly anxiety and depression) and possibly intense concern, tolerance and emotional involvement with their child's symptoms (Garralda & Rangel, 2002). It is important to avoid mistaking the various medical or medication effects of which fatigue can be a feature, and failing to recognize the primary sleep disorders that cause excessive sleepines with which fatigue should not be confused. Clearly, consideration of these possibilities has important implications for choice of advice and treatment.

Garralda ME, Rangel L. (2002). Annotation: Chronic fatigue syndrome in children and adolescents. *J Child Psychol Psychiatry*, **43**, 169–76.

Jackson ML, Bruck D. (2012). Sleep abnormalities in chronic fatigue syndrome/myalgic encephalomyelitis: a review. *J Clin Sleep Med*, **8**, 719–28.

Knight S, Harvey A, Lubitz L *et al.* (2013). Paediatric chronic fatigue syndrome: complex presentations and protracted time to diagnosis. *J Paediatr Child Health*, **49**, 919–24.

Komaroff AL, Cho TA. (2011). Role of infection and neurologic dysfunction in chronic fatigue syndrome. *Semin Neurol*, **31**, 325–37.

Mariman A, Delesie L, Tobback E *et al.* (2013). Undiagnosed and comorbid disorders in patients with presumed chronic fatigue syndrome. *J Psychosom Res*, **75**, 491–6.

Mariman AN, Vogelaers DP, Tobback E *et al.* (2013). Sleep in the chronic fatigue syndrome. *Sleep Med Rev*, **17**, 193–9.

Ohinata J, Suzuki N, Araki A *et al.* (2008). Actigraphic assessment of sleep disorders in children with chronic fatigue syndrome. *Brain Dev*, **30**, 329–33.

Sharpley A, Clements A, Hawton K, Sharpe M. (1997). Do patients with 'pure' chronic fatigue syndrome (neurasthenia) have abnormal sleep? *Psychosom Med*, **59**, 592–6.

Stores G. (1999). Sleep disturbance in chronic fatigue syndrome. *Association of Child Psychology and Psychiatry Occasional Papers* **16**, Chronic Fatigue Syndrome, 13–17.

Stores G, Fry A, Crawford C. (1998), Sleep abnormalities demonstrated by home polysomnography in teenagers with chronic fatigue syndrome. *J Psychosom Res*, **45**, 85–91.

Togo F, Natelson BH, Cherniack NS. *et al.* (2008). Sleep structure and sleepiness in chronic fatigue syndrome with or without coexisting fibromyalgia. *Arthritis Res Ther*, **10**, R56.

Other neurodevelopmental disorders

Traumatic brain injury (TBI)

Studies in various countries indicate that TBI is common (Corrigan *et al.* 2010). For example, in New Zealand about 30% of children, adolescents and young adults experienced at least one TBI, and about a third who experienced a TBI went on to have one or more additional injuries (McKinley *et al.*, 2008). Of the children and adolescents in the United States who annually made almost half a million emergency department visits for TBI, those aged up to 4 years and others aged 15 to 19 years were those most likely to have sustained such an injury (Langlois *et al.*, 2005). TBI can have serious consequences for various aspects of development although the details have yet to be determined (Anderson *et al.*, 2012). The need for further research to help clarify the various imponderables concerning the relationships between TBI and sleep disturbance has been emphasized by Orff *et al.* (2009).

Sleep disturbance

Although there have been various accounts of high rates of sleep disturbance in adults with TBI (Mathias & Alvaro, 2012), such reports about children are relatively few. Although reports concerning adults can be useful in suggesting possibilities in younger patients (Stores & Stores, 2013), there is an obvious need for further, well-designed studies (of patients of all ages) to clarify the many unresolved issues surrounding this topic.

The prevalence of sleep disorders associated with childhood TBI is difficult to estimate but also seems likely to be high. General statements are of limited value because sleep disturbance can be expected to vary with such basic factors as the type of physical trauma (closed head or penetrating), severity (mild, moderate or severe), comorbidity, age of the patient, and when sleep is assessed and re-assessed following the injury. Sleep disturbance may have pre-dated the child's injury but may have worsened subsequently because of the trauma.

Beebe *et al.* (2007) described children with severe TBI as being at increased risk for post-injury sleep problems compared with those with moderate TBI and a control group of children with only an orthopaedic injury. The findings in a prospective study over two years of children and adolescents confirmed a higher rate of sleep disturbance than orthopaedic injury controls (Tham *et al.*, 2012). Sumpter *et al.* (2013) found that moderate to severe childhood TBI was associated with insomnia complaints by parents and children themselves, confirmed by actigraphic findings.

Sleep problems reported by parents or adolescent patients themselves have been described in children and adolescents with mild TBI (Kaufman *et al.*, 2001; Pillar *et al.*, 2003; Milroy *et al.*, 2008). In these studies, subjective complaints have not always been confirmed by objective findings. Doubts have been expressed about the validity of the subjective sleep complaints in view of other instances of subjective–objective disparities such as those reported in other circumstances, including in children with some neurodevelopmental disorders such as ADHD (see earlier). It is possible that traditional objective measures are relatively insensitive to more subtle aspects of sleep physiology such as cyclic alternating pattern (CAP) rates which, if abnormal, might explain some subjective sleep complaints (Parrino et al., 2012).

Sometimes sleep disturbance may be the cause rather than an effect of TBI. Many motor vehicle accidents are due to falling asleep at the wheel for various reasons including sleep loss, sleep apnoea or narcolepsy. Also, some parasomnias (especially those of a violent or otherwise dramatic nature) can result in accidental injury. Avis et al. (2014) found that, on a virtual test of pedestrian safety, children with excessive sleepiness from narcolepsy or idiopathic hypersomnia when compared with healthy controls had impaired decision-making and were twice as likely to be struck by a virtual vehicle.

Types of sleep disturbance

Excessive daytime sleepiness is the sleep problem most consistently described in both adults and children with TBI. Hooper et al. (2004) reported that, in children from infancy to late teens with various degrees of TBI severity, caregivers described excessive sleepiness as a common problem which persisted up to at least 10 months post-injury. In the adult studies reviewed by Stores and Stores (2013), specific sleep disorders likely to explain excessive sleepiness have been sleep apnoea, periodic limb movement disorder, (possibly) narcolepsy and circadian sleep–wake cycle disorders. Fatigue (as distinct from excessive sleepiness but sometimes coexisting with it) has also been described as a consequence of TBI.

Information specifically on childhood insomnia and TBI seems to be lacking although it can be expected in view of the comorbidities and other factors predisposing to sleep disturbance mentioned below. Some studies of adults with TBI report insomnia as common, possibly severe and long-standing, and associated with anxiety, depression and pain, and circadian sleep–wake cycle disorders have also been described (Stores & Stores, 2013).

There is little mention of parasomnias in the literature about childhood TBI and sleep disturbance. However, the adult literature (e.g. Mathias & Alvaro, 2012) refers to a number such as nightmares (to be expected as part of post-traumatic stress disorder), sleepwalking, nocturnal enuresis and REM sleep behaviour disorder. Periodic limb movements in sleep (one of a subset of the parasomnias) has already been mentioned. It is possible that, in at least some instances, such parasomnias (and other sleep problems and disorders) pre-dated the brain injury and, if so, might have been worsened as a result of the insult.

Factors potentially contributing to sleep disturbance

Pathophysiological. The physiological effects of the brain damage inflicted by the injury are fundamental. Damage can occur in 'primary', 'secondary' and 'tertiary' stages over a period of time, each stage involving different pathological processes (Huh & Raghupathi, 2009) possibly giving rise to successive adverse effects including those involving sleep–wake systems. Baumann et al. (2009) have reported a depletion of hypocretin neurons in adult patients with severe TBI which, they suggest, might explain the excessive sleepiness associated with their disorder. Intellectual impairment and inability to communicate effectively, all of which will vary according to the severity of the TBI, may interfere with the learning of good sleep habits or their reacquisition.

Physical comorbidities. Such comorbidities include pain (including headache) which is reported to be common in TBI even with minor injuries (Nampiaparampil, 2008), sleep related breathing problems, post-traumatic epilepsy, mobility problems causing discomfort in bed, blindness (which can give rise to sleep–wake cycle disorders from lack of visual input to the suprachiasmatic nucleus) and nocturnal incontinence.

Psychiatric comorbidities. The serious effects on overall quality of life of TBI in children and adolescents have been reviewed by Di Battista *et al.* (2012). This degree of disruption is likely to have effects on sleep. More specifically, psychiatric conditions such as anxiety states and depression, reported to be common accompaniments of TBI in adults, predispose to sleep problems and, indeed, behavioural and psychiatric states likely to have the same effect have been described in children with TBI. For example, Andrews *et al.* (1998) referred to antisocial and aggressive behaviour, Hooper *et al.* (2004) mentioned personality changes and low frustration intolerance, Max *et al.* (2012) emphasized anxiety and depression, and Karver *et al.* (2012) described ADHD symptoms and anxiety. The last authors and others, such as Kenardy *et al.* (2012) writing about children with TBI and post-traumatic stress disorder, have emphasized the often enduring nature of these psychiatric problems and, therefore, the need for long-term help. Tham *et al.* (2012) sounded a similar note.

Medication effects. The various paediatric medications which might be used as part of the care of children with TBI might include some which can affect sleep and wakefulness. The introduction or increased dosage should be monitored for the possible development or worsening of sleep disturbance.

Parenting. Parents' ability to promote good sleep patterns in their child is likely to be impaired if they are themselves sleep deprived, anxious or depressed, as is likely to be the case if the child is suffering from TBI especially if it is severe and accompanied by various complications (Meltzer & Mindell, 2007). The burden imposed on families of children with TBI has been emphasized by Aitken *et al.* (2009).

Sleep assessment
As part of rehabilitation and continuing care, because of the possible progression of the effects of TBI in the stages described above, reassessment at intervals of a child's sleep (and the other aspects of his condition capable of affecting sleep) is required following the initial assessment.

Aspects of management
The paucity of information about interventions specifically for sleep problems in children with TBI has been pointed out by Galland *et al.* (2012). Some guidance

appropriate for such children may be gained from the limited reports concerning adults. For example, excessive daytime sleepiness (but not fatigue) has been reported to show a positive response to treatment with modafinil (Kaiser *et al.* 2010). Clearly, controlled trials of the use of these various treatments in the TBI context for both adults and children are required. In the meantime, use can be made of the various types of treatment described in Chapter 1 for children's sleep disorders in general. Adequate pain relief is clearly essential. An additional aspect of treatment for sleep disturbance includes education of parents about children's sleep including the importance of the principles of sleep hygiene to encourage good sleep habits. Attention also needs to be given to the possible contributions to sleep disturbance of the factors mentioned above.

Although much has been written about rehabilitation of patients with TBI with otherwise detailed design of rehabilitation programmes, often sleep problems and their consequences and management receive little mention. A proportion of children with TBI may have unmet or unrecognized healthcare needs during the post-injury period, the risk of which is associated with abnormal family functioning according to Slomine *et al.* (2006). As mentioned previously, the neuropathological effects of TBI may change and continue for some time post-injury. Therefore, the children's needs may also alter, and it is important to monitor their recovery comprehensively to ensure that they receive the service that they need (Stancin *et al.*, 2002). This should include correcting any mistaken belief by parents that treatment for their child's sleep disturbance is unlikely to be effective.

Having described the frequency of disturbed behaviour after childhood TBI, Li and Liu (2013) emphasized the importance of long-term follow-up and suggested ways in which such problem behaviour might be reduced. McKinley *et al.* (2012) have emphasized the importance on initial and subsequent assessment of special attention to the impact of TBI on children with an intellectual disability and avoidance of incorrectly attributing TBI symptoms to their pre-existing condition.

Aitken ME, McCarty ML, Slomine BS *et al.* (2009).Family burden after traumatic brain injury in children. *Pediatrics*, **123**, 199–206.

Anderson V, Godfrey C, Rosenfeld JV, Catroppa C *et al.* (2012). 10 years outcome from childhood traumatic brain injury. *Int J Dev Neurosci*, **30**, 217–24.

Andrews TK, Rose FD, Johnson DA. (1998). Social and behavioral effects of traumatic brain injury in children. *Brain Inj*, **12**, 133–8.

Avis KT, Gamble KL, Schwebel DC. (2014). Does excessive daytime sleepiness affect children's pedestrian safety? *Sleep*, **37**, 283–7.

Baumann CR, CR, Bqassetti CL, Valco PO. (2009). Loss of hypocretin (orexin) neurons with traumatic brain injury. *Ann Neurol*, **66**, 555–9.

Beebe DW, Krivitzky L, Wells CT *et al.* (2007). Brief report: parental report of sleep behaviors following moderate or severe pediatric traumatic brain injury. *J Pediatr Psychol*, **32**, 845–50.

Corrigan JD, Selassie AW, Orman JA. (2010). The epidemiology of traumatic brain injury. *J Head Trauma Rehabil*, **25**, 72–80.

Di Battista A, Soo C, Catroppa C, Anderson V. (2012). Quality of life in children and adolescents post-TBI: a systematic review and meta-analysis. *J Neurotrauma*, **29**, 1717–27.

Galland BC, Elder DE, Taylor BJ. (2012). Interventions with sleep outcome for children with cerebral palsy or a post-traumatic brain injury: a systematic review. *Sleep Med Rev*, **16**, 561–73.

Hooper SR, Alexander J, Moore D *et al.* (2004). Caregiver reports of common symptoms in children following traumatic brain injury. *NeuroRehabilitation*, **19**, 175–89.

Huh JW, Raghupathi R. (2009). New concepts in treatment of pediatric traumatic brain injury. *Anesthesiol Clin*, **27**, 213–40.

Kaiser PR, Valco PO, Werth E *et al.* (2010). Modafinil ameliorates excessive daytime sleepiness after traumatic brain injury. *Neurology*, **75**, 1780–5.

Karver CL, Wade SL, Cassedy A *et al.* (2012). Age at injury and long-term behavior problems after traumatic brain injury in young children. *Rehabil Psychol*, **57**, 256–65.

Kaufman Y, Tzischinsky O, Epstein R *et al.* (2001). Long-term sleep disturbances in adolescents after minor head injury. *Pediatr Neurol*, **24**, 129–34.

Kenardy J, Le Brocque R, Hendrikz J. *et al.* (2012). Impact of posttraumatic stress disorder and injury severity on recovery in children with traumatic brain injury. *J Clin Child Adolesc Psychol*, **41**, 5–14.

Langlois JA, Rutland-Brown W, Thomas KE. (2005). The incidence of traumatic brain injury among children in the United Stes: difference by race. *J Head Trauma Rehabil*, **20**, 229–38.

Li L, Liu J. (2013). The effect of pediatric traumatic brain injury on behavioral outcomes: a systematic review. *Dev Med Child Neurol*, **55**, 37–45.

Mathias JL, Alvaro PK. (2012). Prevalence of sleep disturbances, disorders, and problems following traumatic brain injury: a meta-analysis. *Sleep Med*, **13**, 898–905.

Max JE, Wilde EA, Bigler ED *et al.* (2012). Psychiatric disorders after pediatric traumatic brain injury: a prospective, longitudinal, controlled study. *J Neuropsychiatry Clin Neurosci*, **24**, 427–36.

McKinlay A, Grace RC, Horwood LJ *et al.* (2008). Prevalence of traumatic brain injury among children, adolescents and young adults: prospective evidence from a birth cohort. *Brain Inj*, **22**, 175–81.

McKinlay A, McLellan T, Daffue C. (2012). The invisible brain injury: the importance of identifying deficits following brain injury in children with intellectual disability. *NeuroRehabilitation*, **30**, 183–7.

Meltzer LJ, Mindell JA. (2007). Relationship between child disturbance and maternal sleep, mood, and parenting stress: a pilot study. *J Fam Psychol*, **21**, 67–73.

Milroy G, Dorris L, McMillan TM. (2008). Sleep disturbances following mild traumatic brain injury in childhood. *J Pediatr Psychol*, **33**, 242–7.

Nampiaparampil DE. (2008). Prevalence of chronic pain after traumatic brain injury: a systematic review. *JAMA*, **300**, 711–19.

Orff HJ, Ayalon L, Drummond SP. (2009). Traumatic brain injury and sleep disturbance: a review of current research. *J Head Trauma Rehabil*, **24**, 155–65.

Parrino L, Ferri R, Bruni O, Terzano MG. (2012). Cyclic alternating pattern (CAP): the marker of sleep instability. *Sleep Med Rev*, **16**, 27–45.

Pillar G, Averbooch E, Katz N *et al.* (2003). Prevalence and risk of sleep disturbances in adolescents after minor head injury. *Pediatr Neurol*, **29**, 131–5.

Slomine Bs, McCarthy ML, Ding R. (2006). Health care utilization and needs after pediatric traumatic brain injury. *Pediatrics*, **117**, e663–74.

Stancin T, Drotar D, Taylor HG *et al.* (2002). Health-related quality of life of children and adolescents after traumatic brain injury. *Pediatrics*, **109**, E34.

Stores G, Stores R. (2013). Sleep disorders in children with traumatic brain injury: a case of serious neglect. *Dev Med Child Neurol*, **55**, 797–805.

Sumpter RE, Dorris L, Kelly T, McMillan TM. (2013). Pediatric sleep difficulties after moderate–severe traumatic brain injury. *J Int Neuropsychol Soc*, **19**, 829–34.

Tham SW, Palermo TM, Vavilala MS *et al.* (2012). The longitudinal course, risk factors, and impact of sleep disturbances in children with traumatic brain injury. *J Neurotrauma*, **29**, 154–61.

Cerebral palsy (CP)

CP is defined as a group of permanent disorders of the development of movement and posture that are attributed to non-progressive disturbances that occurred in the developing foetal or infant brain. The motor disorders of the condition are often accompanied by disturbances of sensation, perception, cognition, communication and behaviour, by epilepsy, and by secondary musculoskeletal problems (Rosenbaum *et al.*, 2007). Diverse aspects of CP (not just type of motor abnormality) need to be taken into account in classifying CP for practical clinical purposes. It follows that generalizations about children with CP are rarely justified. Overall prevalence is in the order of 2 to 2.5 per 1000 live births.

Sleep disturbance
Consistently, sleep problems are reported to be common in children with CP (Kotagal *et al.*, 1994; Newman *et al.*, 2006; Simard-Tremblay *et al.*, 2011; Romeo *et al.*, 2014).

Types of sleep disturbance
In the survey by Newman *et al.* (2006) of children with CP, the most common sleep problems were difficulty settling to sleep, staying asleep and waking up in the morning, as well as sleep related breathing disorders. Correlates of these problems were spastic quadriplegic and dyskinetic CP, and also severe visual impairment which is likely to predispose to abnormalities in circadian sleep–wake rhythm. On the basis of sleep questionnare results, Elsayed *et al.* (2013) reported high rates of insomnia and bruxism in preschool children with CP, and sleep disordered breathing, nightmares, sleep talking and excessive daytime sleepiness in those of school age. In the sleep questionnaire study by Romeo *et al.* (2014), 42% of children with CP were found to have an abnormal score for at least one of the following types of sleep disturbance: insomnia, sleep related breathing disorder, arousal disorder, excessive daytime sleepiness, and excessive sweating during sleep. Highest rates of sleep disturbance were seen in the dyskinetic subgroup with equal rates in the other types of CP. Intellectual disability, active epilepsy, behavioural/psychiatric disturbance and high levels of disturbance in gross motor function were associated with an abnormal total sleep score.

Excessive daytime sleepiness can be expected to be a prominent problem in view of the high rate of epilepsy in children with CP, which Pruitt and Tsai (2009) reported to be over 70% in those with intellectual disability. Sleep related breathing disorders in children with CP may well consist of combinations of obstructive and central apnoea or hypoventilation, often of severe degree (Kotagal *et al.*, 1994). The findings of Sandella *et al.* (2011) illustrate the impairment in quality of life that can be caused by such sleep disturbances in children with CP.

Factors potentially contributing to sleep disturbance

Pathophysiological. In view of the diversity and severity of CP, and the structures and mechanisms involved in sleep and wakefulness that might be affected, it is not surprising that sleep disturbance is so common and can take the various forms mentioned above. Intellectual disability, and its degree, vary with the type of CP with an overall prevalence in the order of 50%. This, and also poor communication skills, can interfere with learning to sleep well.

Physical comorbidities. Pruitt and Tsai (2009) and Simard-Tremblay *et al.* (2011) have discussed medical factors associated with the development of sleep problems in children with CP. As in the case of other neurodevelopmental disorders, the relevance of epilepsy is convincing as a contributory factor in sleep disturbance in children with CP (Carlsson *et al.*, 2003). Similarly, the high rate of cortical visual impairment is seen as a risk factor for sleep problems, as is pain or discomfort from abnormal muscular tone, as well as the repeated attention from their parents that severely disabled children might need at night. The effects on mental health and quality of life of recurrent musculoskeletal pain in children with CP were discussed by Ramstad *et al.* (2012). Contractures and other orthopaedic problems, for which postural equipment is used, are other sleep disruptive problems in those children who are severely physically disabled (Hill *et al.*, 2009).

Psychiatric comorbidities. In keeping with other reports, Bjorgaas *et al.* (2013) described high rates of various types of psychiatric problems in their group of children with CP compared with children in the general population. These consisted of emotional problems, conduct problems, attention deficit hyperactivity-type behaviours, and difficulties in their relationships with their peers (the measures used in their study did not include assessment for autism spectrum disorders). Overall, 57% met criteria for some form of psychiatric disorder, all of which would predispose to sleep disturbance as discussed in Chapter 3. Similar findings regarding behavioural problems in school age children with CP have been reported by Brossard-Racine *et al.* (2012), with such problems being particularly associated with parental stress.

Medication. Possible effects on sleep and wakefulness of drugs for physical or psychiatric disorders need to be considered in the usual way.

Parenting. In view of the problems for parents that can be posed by CP, Simard-Tremblay *et al.* (2011) rightly emphasize the parental difficulties that can be associated with childhood CP which increase the likelihood of sleep disturbance in both their child and also themselves (Wayte *et al.*, 2012). Romeo *et al.* (2010)

provided insights into the effects on the quality of life of parents of children with CP, including their child's behaviour.

Assessment

As usual, this needs to be comprehensive concerning the detection and diagnosis of sleep disturbance and possible contributory factors. It is important to screen children with CP for psychiatric problems and to assess the impact on the family of the child's condition.

Aspects of the management of sleep disturbance

Behavioural and pharmacological treatment possibilities, similar to those for other neurodevelopmental disorders where the sleep disturbance is of multifactorial origin, are considered by Simard-Tremblay *et al.* (2011), and Grigg-Damberger and Stanley (2011) discuss treatment options for sleep related breathing disorders in CP. Although, the evidence base for these various treatments is often limited (Galland *et al.*, 2012), it is appropriate to seriously consider their use in the individual child. Mol *et al.* (2012) considered ways of helping parents in their use of night orthoses for children with severe physical disabilities likely to affect their sleep. In their study of children with hemiplegia, Goodman and Graham (1996) stressed the need ideally for the provision of comprehensive mental health services for this group of children. Without early intervention or preventative measures, their psychiatric problems may persist long-term (Goodman, 1998). The importance of detailed mental health screening and careful follow-up for children with CP was also stressed by Bjorgaas *et al.* (2013).

Bjorgaas HM, Elgen I, Boe T, Hysing M. (2013). Mental health in children with cerebral palsy: does screening capture the complexity? *Scientic World Journal*, April 3, 468402.

Brossard-Racine M, Hall N, Majnemer A *et al.* (2012). Behavioural problems in school age children with cerebral palsy. *Eur J Paediatr Neurol*, **16**, 35–41.

Carlsson M, Hagberg G, Olsson I. (2003). Clinical and aetiological aspects of epilepsy in children with cerebral palsy. *Dev Med Child Neurol*, **45**, 371–6.

Elsayed RM, Hasanein BM, Sayyah HE *et al.* (2013). Sleep assessment of children with cerebral parsy: using a validated sleep questionnaire. *Ann Indian Acad Neurol*, **16**, 455.

Galland BC, Elder DE, Taylor BJ. (2012). Interventions with sleep outcome for children with cerebral palsy or a post-traumatic brain injury: a systematic review. *Sleep Med Rev*, **16**, 561–73.

Goodman R. (1998). The longitudinal stability of psychiatric problems in children with hemiplegia. *J Child Psychol Psychiatry*, **39**, 347–54.

Goodman R, Graham P. (1996). Psychiatric problems in children with hemiplegia: cross sectional epidemiological survey. *BMJ*, **312** (7038), 1065–9.

Grigg-Damberger M, Stanley JJ. Children with intellectual disabilities and/or cerebral palsy. In: Kothare SV, Kotagal S, eds. *Sleep in Childhood Neurological Disorders*. New York: demos Medical 2011. 254–5.

Hill CM, Parker RC, Allen P, Paul A, Padoa KA. (2009). Sleep quality and respiratory function in children with severe cerebral palsy using night-time postural equipment: a pilot study. *Acta Paediatr*, **98**, 1809–14.

Kotagal S, Gibbons VP, Stith JA. (1994). Sleep abnormalities in patients with severe cerebral palsy. *Dev Med Child Neurol*, **36**, 304–11.

Mol EM, Monbaliu E, Ven M, Vergote M, Prinzie P. (2012). The use of night orthroses in cerebral palsy treatment: sleep disturbance in children and parental burden or not? *Res Dev Disabil*, **33**, 341–9.

Newman CJ, O'Regan M, Hensey O. (2006). Sleep disorders in children with cerebral palsy. *Dev Med Child Neurol*, **48**, 564–8.

Pruitt DW, Tsai T. (2009). Common medical comorbidities associated with cerebral palsy. *Phys Med Rehabil Clin N Am*, **20**, 453–67.

Ramstad K, Jahnsen R, Skjeldal OH, Diseth TH. (2012). Mental health, health related quality of life and recurrent musculoskeletal pain in children with cerebral palsy 8–18 years old. *Disabil Rehab*, **34**, 1589–95.

Romeo DM, Brogna C, Quintiliani M *et al.* (2014). Sleep disorders in children with cerebral palsy: neurodevelopmental and behavioral correlates. *Sleep Med*, **15**, 213–18.

Romeo DM, Cioni M, Distefano A *et al.*(2010). Quality of life in parents of children with cerebral palsy: is it influenced by the child's behaviour? *Neuropediatrics*, **41**, 121–6.

Rosenbaum P, Paneth N, Leviton A *et al.* (2007). A report: the definition and classification of cerebral palsy April 2006. *Dev Med Child Neurol*, **109**, 8–14.

Sandella DE, O'Brien LM, Shank LK, Warchausky SA. (2011). Sleep and quality of life in children with cerebral palsy. *Sleep Med*, **12**, 252–6.

Simard-Tremblay E, Constantin E, Gruber R, Brouillette RT, Shevell M. (2011). Sleep in children with cerebral palsy: a review. *J Child Neurol*, **26**, 1303–10.

Wayte S, McCaughey E, Holley S, Annaz D, Hill CM. (2012). Sleep problems in children with cerebral palsy and their relationship with maternal sleep and depression. *Acta Paediatr*, **101**, 618–23.

Developmental coordination disorder (DCD)

The review by Zwicker *et al.* (2012) describes DCD as present in 5–6% of school-aged children and characterized by motor coordination difficulties which significantly interfere with daily living activities or academic achievement. Difficulties are encountered with tasks that call for fine and/or gross motor skills including hand-eye coordination, and balance and agility. Sleep aspects of the condition have received little attention, but it has been associated with various problems and conditions each capable of affecting sleep adversely such as anxiety and attention deficit hyperactivity disorder (Barnett & Wiggs, 2012). These authors' own preliminary study produced evidence to suggest that, indeed, a group of children with DCD had rates of sleep disturbance in excess of those of typically developing children, particularly in the form of bedtime resistance, a mixture of parasomnia-like phenomena, and also daytime sleepiness. This last feature might be related to comorbid obesity which, in turn, may be linked to avoidance of physical exercise (Cairney *et al.*, 2005; Cairney *et al.*, 2012).

Barnett AL, Wiggs L. (2012). Sleep behaviour in children with developmental co-ordination disorder. *Child Care Health Dev*, **38**, 403–11.

Cairney J, Hay JA, Faught BE, Hawes R. (2005). Developmental coordination disorder and overweight and obesity in children aged 9–14 y. *Int J Obes (Lond)*, **29**, 369–72.

Cairney J, Kwan MY, Hay JA, Faught BE. (2012). Developmental coordination disorder, gender, and body weight: examining the impact of participation in active play. *Res Dev Disabil*, **33**, 1566–73.

Zwicker JG, Missiuna C, Harris SR, Boyd LA. (2012). Developmental coordination disorder: a review and update. *Eur J Paediatr Neurol*, **16**, 573–81.

Envoi

The introductory remarks at the start of this book include expressions of regret that, despite the convincing evidence that persistently disturbed sleep is likely to have significantly unwelcome psychological, physical and social consequences in anyone at any age, sleep and its disorders are a seriously neglected topic in the training of healthcare professionals as well as health education for the general public. Matters are improving to some extent, but the pace is slow. Consequently, many opportunities are being lost for the prevention and treatment of the ill effects of disordered sleep.

This is particularly unfortunate in the case of individuals already disadvantaged in other ways. Children with neurodevelopmental disorders are a clear case in point. It is not over-dramatic to say that there is an urgent need for much more attention being given to the sleep disturbances common in children with the types of conditions reviewed in the last chapter. This review clearly demonstrates that, at present, information about these conditions is incomplete and, indeed, lacking for many other neurodevelopmental disorders. As stated earlier, because the scientific merit is variable from one published study to another, the conclusions drawn are often necessarily provisional, but they raise important possibilities for consideration in clinical practice as well as suggesting the many areas requiring further research.

The contrast between the increasing attention given to genetic aspects in the neurodevelopmental disorders field and that paid to sleep aspects of these conditions is difficult to over-state. Correcting this imbalance is not an easy task because of the aetiological complexity of sleep disturbance in children with a neurodevelopmental disorder compared with most typically developing children. This review is meant to emphasize the multifactorial nature of factors (pathophysiological, physical or psychiatric comorbidities, medication and parenting factors) which may collectively conspire to cause the sleep disturbances that are commonplace in neurologically compromised children. This potential complexity has clear implications for the assessment and care of the individual child. However, the integrated multidisciplinary contributions ideally required can only be achieved with improved knowledge (on the part of the professionals and parents involved) of sleep disorders and their complexity in such children. This book is aimed at making a contribution towards that end.

Index

Printed in the United States
by Baker & Taylor Publisher Services